LYME
WITH A TWIST

A Path to Triumph Over Chronic Infection

LYME WITH A TWIST

A Path to Triumph Over Chronic Infection

LOWELL MILLER

To contact the author, please write to:
lowellmiller@mail.com

Mr. Lyme sculpture by Lowell Miller
Cover design by Elizabeth Cline

A PRINT PROJECT BOOK

ISBN: 978-0-9840938-5-4

CONTENTS

Lyme with a Twist 1

August 2020: To the ER 3

August 1982: Bitten—The Story Begins, Then Goes 11

2002: Stress Triggers a Fire Down Below 17

2002: Doctor 1: A First Mainstream Doctor 23

2002: First Neurologist 27

2003: Driven to the Alternatives 29

2003: I Meet Ketek 35

2012: Monster Face 39

A Few Things about Lyme 45

Ketek Has a Story of Its Own 49

2017: Down the Research Rabbit Hole 57

2020: COVID Begins 69

Onward to the Hospital! 73

Finding a Top Guy to Help Me 79

2021: After the Dam Has Burst, a Flood 85

Finally, a Definitive Diagnosis 95

End of 2022: Treatment Failure 107

2023: The Twist 111

Into Herb World 121

2024: A Twist on the Twist 135

My Takeaways and a Notion of Infectious Disease 139

2024: My "Recipe" 143

About the Author 146

LYME WITH A TWIST

In the forests that surround our house live the deer, as they always have. We're reminded of this every summer evening, when a small herd comes to browse the broad green lawn at dusk. As they pass by low branches and bushes, *Ixodes* ticks that have been lurking on twig ends or leaves leap on for a ride on those strong, caramel-colored backs, traveling as far as the deer may roam. No one watches; it's all just behind the screen of busy nature. Ticks spread silently through the forests on deer or, for a shorter ride, on mice, squirrels, chipmunks, raccoons.

The deer seem sweet as they saunter into our yard. Their little tails flick quickly at flies. They have an innocent, almost beggarly look in their large brown eyes. They seem to want to chat. Still, I can't help myself. I hate them. I want to run after them shouting and banging pans.

But for the deer, I would not have lived my adult life with Lyme disease; I'd not feel this compulsion to set forth the actual experience of Lyme, the inner misery and the frustrating experience of trying to cure it. It occupies and clouds both outer and inner life. This illness is felt within, incessantly and mercilessly. Yes, there are uprising headline symptoms, take-me-to-the-ER symptoms, but most consistently it's a disease of deterioration, an undermining undertow slowing down the body and the mind to a point of debility, removing the life from life, without end.

There are statistics you can cite. There are metabolic processes with scientific names at work here, the busy biology of the body. But I'm not a doctor; I'm not a research scientist. I hide behind no white coat. And I'm not, according to my lawyers, "offering medical advice or prescription, and nothing in this book should be considered medical advice."

Here I recount my life with Lyme, hoping to let fellow sufferers see that you're not alone. My disease trip ended in a surprise, what I can only call a "twist." I can't say it will work the same for everyone—this illness manifests differently in different people, and has many mysteries. I spent the time to draw many scenes of its appearance because I hope it will be helpful.

AUGUST 2020:
To the ER

Visualize me in August of 2020 all alone under the sun, post-retirement but feeling energetic, playing tennis against a ball machine on a beat-up old court that came with our property. It was so hot then, steamy hot; heat waves rippled up off the blacktop, wobbling the air. Tennis had become my COVID outdoor hobby; nearly every day I'd go out and practice. My serve was definitely coming along.

In general it was a positive period; feeling expansive and healthy, the facets of my life lining up harmonically. I'd recently sold my investment management business. For many years that company had forced my deeper passions of writing and sculpture down to a low simmer; now my time was finally open for what I wanted, when I wanted. (Free at last!) Even the pandemic was a plus; a readymade excuse to stay home for activities that awakened my central being.

Though past 70, I was optimistic and surprised at how young and alive I felt every morning.

Anyway, on this hot day, sweat was flowing from every pore and streaming into my eyes. But racquet hit after hit, the sun on my head was still friendly, no matter the extra heat. In a quiet moment I gathered my breath, considered whether my follow-through was precise enough, and casually walked up to the net for ball pickup. All normal. However, as I bent down to grab a loose ball, I missed the grab. Odd. I tried again, getting lower and closer to it . . . but still missed. Without warning I found myself going yet lower, slowly sinking down onto the court, knees buckling. Instinctively I reached for the net, hooking my fingers in it to stay upright. But I couldn't lift. I became helpless, melting in slow motion, unable to yank myself back up, my fingers slipping off the netting. Falling into a feeling of terror. I hollered for my son (who'd returned home to live with us during the pandemic), but my voice didn't work right, emerging from my chest rather than my lips, which could not form words. Inside I had the feeling I was a braying donkey. A large braying donkey booming out over the yard in the hot summer sun, calling for help. Before my son could arrive I went completely down, and then out. Fade to blackness. All black. I was gone.

Though still short-circuited, I had a vague sense that there were people around me. I could hear unfamiliar voices. As my eyes briefly opened, I saw that they'd moved me and were loading my limp body onto a gurney, sliding it into the local rescue squad ambulance. Someone said, "He's stroking out." Someone else said, "Oh, that's a bad one." (Note to self: Inform the rescue squad folks that even an apparently unconscious patient can still hear.) Then I couldn't physically open my eyes and didn't really know what was happening, though I heard them speaking gibberish before fading back into blackness again. But wait . . . it couldn't actually be me stroking out?!

Now conscious in the ER, I could see that four or five staff surrounded me. They talked to a high-rank doctor who loomed on a mounted TV monitor. No, even though I commanded it with my mind, my left hand could not rise. All agreed, I had to go "upstairs." It would be the first time in my life I'd gone upstairs, except as a visitor.

Eventually I learned that this apparent stroke may have looked like a stroke, but it wasn't. As I'll explain later, it was a consequence of Lyme bacteria that had been slowly but surely accumulating within me for decades—like scum on the lily pond of my brain. The microbial colonization had at last reached a moment of overload, a figurative and literal tipping point. I'd had other Lyme-related events over the years, but this was the most radical of episodes. Nothing before had put me in the hospital.

With little else to do in that sterile bed apart from resting and watching crummy daytime TV, I worked my memory back to the beginning. It's a melancholy narrative; the story of life in conflict with a tenacious bacteria living like a fattening leech on my brain. There was little help to pry it off; I had to find my own path toward relief. Even now, more than four decades after the "discovery" of Lyme, no MD can offer a targeted cure that's been proven effective in most chronic patients. I had the bad luck to be bitten in 1982, when Lyme disease was virtually unknown—and therefore my case went undiagnosed and untreated for many years, for decades. You can be symptom-free for that long and not know you're actually ill until it's too late.

So who am I, and why would I interest you? I am a detailed case study. A study of how Lyme can cohabit in its host, appearing and disappearing and reappearing with long breaks in between. Mine is one story of how it can enter your central nervous system and produce a myriad of symptoms mimicking many other illnesses—

though they are Lyme, not those other conditions. I write this up, in part because there aren't any published studies of a Lyme case that's lasted over 40 years, and in part because I finally did find a kind of salvation despite a lack of formal or official guidance—and I want to share it. Medical science has little to say or do about a case so long, or even a shorter one that's become "chronic."

Illness happens to a subject. This case is about more than just a bag of infected biomass. I was living a life (though impinged) all the while. The focus is not just disease, then, but disease in the context of living. Living and persisting. So I show this disease tangibly embedded in my life as it unfolded, the life in which my parasite has lived. If you're interested in Lyme, you might find the resolution at which I arrived—a resolution outside of traditional medical practice—to be something real, and worth knowing.

▪ ▪ ▪

In the late 1970s and early 1980s, Lyme disease was not a topic of conversation or concern, even in the Northeast, where it eventually became endemic. No one had heard of it. It did not arise spontaneously or arrive suddenly on a ship from Europe. It had been present in this country for a while—and in Europe for hundreds of years, perhaps even dating from before the Ice Age, according to archaeological evidence—but no one had heard of it. It had not been seen under a microscope; it had not been named. No one knew what it was, or even *that* it was.

In June of 1980, I visited my friend Howard, a film director for TV commercials. He was also a potter and had a studio on his property in Westchester, as well as a share in a vacation house on Block Island—two spots that we know today, but didn't know then, are major areas of infestation with the black-legged tick *Ixodes*, which is the primary carrier of *Borrelia burgdorferi* (the bug that causes Lyme) through its bite. Add a pair of pet German shepherd dogs to the mix, and Howard was almost destined to get bitten just as soon as the biting had begun. This was the first moment when I saw firsthand what Lyme disease can do—though the concept of Lyme hadn't really entered my brain yet; it was still an alien and abstract idea. It was something I'd never had and couldn't imagine I ever would.

In symptoms, Howard's manifestation was mainly arthritic or joint-centered. He'd gone from specialist to specialist for months in Westchester and New York City to get his debilitating arthritis diagnosed and cured. But every rheumatologist he saw said, "No, you don't have arthritis." Arthritis has a special signature of state and symptoms, with bone deterioration visible in medical imaging, and Howard didn't have what they'd need to see to make a diagnosis. All he had to offer was intense soreness and pain in nearly every joint!

When I came by, his wife sent me to go see him in his studio. I was shocked. He was pacing around the studio over and over, around and around the studio, until I finally got a good look at his face. It was all ... twisted. One eye was shut, and his mouth was dropping steeply to one side. The only face I'd ever seen like that was on a movie monster.

This was Bell's palsy, an infection and inflammation of the seventh facial nerve (which controls the eye and mouth muscles), mimicking the look of stroke. It turns out that Bell's palsy is a fairly predictable manifestation or symptom of Lyme, but at the time Howard didn't know that, and was sunk in terror that he was doomed at age 38 to an ugly and distorted monster face for the rest of his life, to go along with his whole-body joint aching and pain.

His panic increased over the days, days filled with trips from doctor to doctor. Finally, after months of anxiety, there was word of a research effort at Yale that had started a few years prior, and a ray of hope. Howard followed that ray to the initial group of doctors in New Haven who were working on the problem, and he finally received some help that reduced his symptoms, though it was far from a cure.

A little Lyme Wiki:

In 1975, the Connecticut State Health Department received complaints from artist and mother Polly Murray, a resident of Lyme, Connecticut. Two of her children had been diagnosed with juvenile rheumatoid arthritis, but she knew of many others in the area with similar symptoms.

An epidemic intelligence officer from the health department brought in Dr. Allen Steere, a rheumatologist at Yale, to investigate. Steere had been at the Centers for Disease Control (CDC) in the Epidemic Intelligence Service, a CDC program set up in the 1950s to track epidemics worldwide. Steere called each family on a list Ms. Murray had given him including 39 children, and he found an additional 12 adults suffering from what was diagnosed by local doctors as juvenile rheumatoid arthritis.

A quarter of the people Steere interviewed remembered getting a strange, spreading skin rash before experiencing any other symptoms. In a sort of coincidence not uncommon in the world of science, a European doctor happened to be visiting Yale at the time, and he pointed out that the rash was similar to one frequently encountered in northern Europe and known to be associated with tick bites. Most of the rashes were found somewhere on the torso, suggesting a crawling vector rather than a flying one or a spider, but most patients didn't remember being bitten.

Over the next year Steere began testing blood from disease victims for specific antibodies against 38 known tick-transmitted diseases and 178 other arthropod-transmitted viruses. Not one came out positive.

Steere then learned about the work of the Swedish dermatologist Arvid Afzelius, who in 1909 had described an expanding, ring-like lesion and speculated that it was caused by the bite of an *Ixodes* tick. The rash described by Afzelius was later named erythema migrans. Research in Europe had found that erythema migrans responded to penicillin, suggesting that the cause was bacterial, not viral. Yet no microorganisms could be found in fluid from the joints of Lyme disease patients. This is still true today: the bacteria that causes Lyme is almost impossible to detect in the fluids of the host. Only antibodies to it produced by the immune system are available for detection.

The recognition that the patients in the United States had erythema migrans led to the recognition that "Lyme arthritis" was one manifestation of the same tick-borne disease known in Europe. The syndrome first found in and around Lyme and Old Lyme, Connecticut, came to be called "Lyme arthritis" and later "Lyme disease." As time went on, researchers realized that neurological Lyme (Lyme neuroborreliosis), infection of the cerebrospinal fluid, was just as likely as infection located at the joints.

Without much of a clue about how to deal with the disease, the Yale doctors threw any likely broad-spectrum antibiotics at it. There was nothing newly developed to specifically target *Borrelia burgdorferi*—the culprit bacteria—and there still is not. This would be the place for a rant on the fact that antibiotics aren't big money makers for the major drug companies, so they don't bother—well, that's the rant right there.

AUGUST 1982:
Bitten—The Story Begins, Then Goes Quiet

Around the time Howard came down with his infection, I was living on a farm with my then partner in Dutchess County, New York. Today we know Dutchess County was to become one of the nation's hot spots for Lyme in the ensuing years. That makes sense: lots of open space for the deer on which the *Borrelia*-carrying *Ixodes* tick likes to travel about, and few hunters. This is actually one of the reasons why Lyme and the ticks that carry it have exploded in recent times. Deer have proliferated in rural and semi-rural places due to the lack of predators, including hunters. Upon the hides of deer, ticks travel hither and yon, landing in fields and bushes, hanging at the tips of leaves, awaiting the nearby passing of a warm-blooded mammal for their next meal, in an anticipatory state that students of the tick call *questing*. Their quest ends in a ride on the static electric charge that any mammal exhibits, surfing a kind of electrostatic wave into an upcoming meal of blood.

In those days we never worried about ticks of any kind, or how they traveled. It was not a part of consciousness. No long pants tucked into socks. No DEET or permethrin on the shoes. No long-sleeved shirts in summer. No languid baths in which every inch of skin was touched and checked by you or your partner. No second thoughts about running into the bushes to retrieve an errant football or new puppy.

Our farmhouse was surrounded by cornfields cultivated by a tenant farmer. So to get from the house out to my studio and home office in the barn, I kicked down a path through the corn, and if I wanted to walk to the seasonal stream that ran alongside the property, I pushed through another path. At dusk, at least a dozen deer made evening nests in their own trampled corn, and you could see dark splotches on the rolling hillside where they lay. The late 1960s were not dead yet. We'd play rock and roll on a boom box and dance in the flattened cornfield areas, high on the marijuana we'd grown atop an old horse manure pile behind the barn—a spot where the deer happily pruned the plants back and made them strong (!). Did I ever wear a shirt on a warm summer day then? No. Did I ever wear long pants? No. Did I ever do a tick check? A *what*?

In 1982 my partner decided she needed to take her daughter, who'd been having trouble adjusting socially in the local school, to a better and more congenial school in New York City. So in July they took an apartment and temporarily moved down there, leaving me with her adolescent son and older daughter. I didn't really mind; I was busy as always with projects in publishing, financial business, and art. July rolled into August. It was deep summer, the sky was painterly blue, and the corn was beginning to mature. Hawks were circling overhead on the thermals. Poplars swayed rhythmically at the edge of the field in periodic breezes. There was no traffic on the roads. I played in a men's soccer league two evenings a week and trained in the martial art of aikido for three. I cut firewood. I built shelves for my office out of clear pine from plans in a magazine. I tended the potted plants when they grew faster than the deer could chew them down. I wrote poetry at dusk. Crickets and tree frogs chanted a call-and-response symphony in the clear dark nights, a constant, syncopated rhythm as if the crowd of them were actually marching to a destination somewhere off in the blackness. It was a good summer in the country.

One day in August, I started to feel hot, way beyond the outside temperature. All of me felt hot, and my head was burning. (Bear in mind that at this point I was just in my mid-30s and still innocent in terms of registering symptoms and knowing what to do to take care of myself. I didn't think to go to a doctor, because of course I didn't have a doctor.) The heat did not let up. My temples began to sweat, and then my whole body began oozing sweat, so much so that I had to take off my clothes and find something dry. Then I soaked the bed and had to change the sheets. (*Hmm, where are the clean sheets?*) Soon the new sheets were wet, too, and I had to change them again. Then I became cold, icy cold, chilled and shaking in every part, no matter that the outside temperature was in the 90s. Then hot again, with profound sweats again. Then shaking chills. Then more fever. Changing the wet sheets again, then changing them yet again. Next I felt a strong buzzing throughout my body, then chills, putting on a ski parka, then the sweats returned. Over and over. *Can I get up for some food? No, I can't get up. Too dizzy ... too dizzy, dizzy.*

I lay like that in bed, sweating and freezing, freezing and sweating, day after day, for some three weeks. I reached a point where it seemed impossible to go on. *Let me go!* I nearly prayed.

Wow, I thought, *this is some kind of flu!* At one point I looked down at my naked body, glistening with sweat. There was a large red rash on both inner thighs.

Now, today anyone living in the county would know: "flu" at the wrong time of year, strong and deep fevers, red rash at the same time—*get to the doctor, you've got Lyme!* But this was 1982. Lyme had barely been "discovered" by the crew at Yale at that point, and the information had hardly trickled into the general population, even to doctors. Today there's a Lyme article featured in every town weekly paper or on the local TV station each spring. Back then, nobody knew. Nobody talked about it. No celebrities announced on social media that they had it. None of your everyday friends had gotten it. Nobody thought a summer flu was strange. Nobody knew what it was.

As an early adopter, I had no sense that something special might be happening to my health. And so I just rested, beaten up by the weeks of fevers and chills—comforted only by the small mercy that I worked from home and didn't have to trudge out in the world for a job. I rested for several months. No early antibiotic or any other kind of treatment. Yet I was only 34 at the time, with a still-young and robust immune system and healthy body that fought back against what I now know were the invaders. Actually, I don't recall ever being sick for more than a few days at any point in my life up until then. I rested to move past the fatigue and weakness and headaches that followed the fevers. I relied on the body's natural ability to heal. Ah, youth! Before too long I was out playing soccer again. Boom!

Those acute symptoms faded over the next months, as a flu might, but I did have one strange residual: whenever I was depleted or especially tired, it felt as if there were bugs crawling under the skin of my arms. I know, or I think I know, there were not really bugs crawling under my skin. But the sensation would arise, a feeling that told me to take a nap, or go to bed. I recognized it right away. *It's the bugs,* I'd tell myself. Recall, at this time Lyme was essentially unknown. Could my body, my body and brain, have been creating a metaphor for what was really going on?

I picked up my life where it had left off, writing and producing books and articles, honing some skills as a stock investor, sculpting, studying aikido with some top teachers who happened to live in the area, starting an investment research firm with a friend who was a computer scientist (that occupation was hardly known in the early 1980s, believe it or not), raising the family, eventually leaving my partner, having love affairs; overall an exciting and energetic life. But I had little stamina. I'd go all out for an activity or event and then feel the bugs again, and flu-like sensations of weakness, perhaps with head heat—my signal to exit stage left for the bedroom and recover in sleep. I came to identify myself as "a fairly healthy guy with a weak immune system." Turns out I couldn't have been more wrong. The immune apparatus was so strong that it suppressed the relentless but silent growth of *Borrelia burgdorferi* for some *20 years* until obvious radical symptoms emerged.

Borrelia is known to be slow growing. It's also an obligate parasite, which means it needs a host to live in. You won't find it on the kitchen counter or on a toilet seat. It needs the warm, nutritious Caribbean of a mammal's blood and soft tissues to make a home, a long-term home. *Borrelia* wants to thrive on the glucose in your blood, and it grows tenaciously, persistently, like algae or moss or rust. A living thing, it wants to live; it doesn't want to kill you. If it didn't reveal its presence, you wouldn't think to do anything about it. The first two decades after my big bite weren't marked by constant, acute symptoms, but the disease was working by stealth—a continuing presence of Borrelia in my system, gradually occupying my fluids and tissues at a rate just slow enough to avoid triggering urgent and loud immune-system alarms. The closest I'd ever come until 2002 to linking present feelings to the past bite were inexplicable bouts of fatigue and the recurrent but intermittent "bugs" under my skin, reminding me of that monumental summer "flu."

2002:

Stress Triggers a Fire Down Below

By 2002, I was founder and head guy of a solid and growing boutique investment management firm, with institutions, advisors, hedge funds, and high-net-worth individuals as clients. After beginning as a research company, we started managing funds in 1991 with no assets under management (though we did still have a research business) and no track record, but within 10 years we were a recommended manager on the advisory platforms of big firms like Morgan Stanley, UBS, Ameriprise, Citicorp, etc. I know this may read like a big jump cut in the medical biography, but from 1984 to 2002 there was little distinct or apparent Lyme action to hold me back; during that time the business evolved, bit by bit, one foot in front of the other. We grew slowly, even as the *Borrelia* was doing the same. The days built up into an enterprise, and *Borrelia* was, at that point, just along for the ride. I had plenty of energy, although I was still subject to sudden and inexplicable bouts of fatigue. My wife tells me I would sometimes fall asleep at dinner in the middle of a conversation.

In any event, the prior year (2001) was one of high stress in the business, and not because it was the moment the tech bubble burst—we didn't invest in those kinds of stocks, only in the most conservative dividend-paying types, which were unscathed. It was the people, my employees and partners, that cranked me up. Business can be fun, but dealing with and depending on people, not so much. Stress interacts with health, a much deeper connection than we usually assume, until the stress induces a breakthrough. Business stress did soon enough wind up triggering the "bugs," tricking them into showing themselves.

Flash back to the late 1970s, more than 20 years prior: I published a book on technical analysis of stocks called *The Momentum-Gap Method* (G. P. Putnam's Sons, 1978), providing a rule-based system for stock investing that I'd developed—during many late nights poring over stock charts out in my barn—and implemented successfully, especially with options. This caught the eye of John C., an investment newsletter publisher who got in touch with me to write one of his publications. I worked with him for a few years, earning what at the time was a nice sum for writing five or so pages each month. Since it was before the age of email—even faxing was a new thing—every month I'd drive down an hour or two with my pages and meet with him, in an office downstairs in his Westchester split-level (where the wet bar used to be!), sometimes having lunch with him and his quiet wife (a piano teacher). He seemed like a solid guy, on the school board, coach of a high school soccer team, natural father of three, adoptive father of three more, with a rotating cast of four or five foster children. He could make a team of his own, right in the house.

One of his newsletters specialized in very small-cap stocks. Our firm didn't have any expertise in this type, so, in 2001, I called on him—reviving our connection after 15 years—to become the sub-advisor for us in starting a small-cap portfolio—our first "product" expansion. Because we had a growing string of advisors who trusted us and our judgment, and because there is a dearth of small-cap managers, accounts started flowing to us right away. We made a partnership with him, in which he'd pick the stocks and we'd do the back office and trading and marketing. Good for both (!). Having seen his newsletter picks over the years, I thought he'd do well. Also, anyone signing up for a small-cap strategy knows they're getting hot sauce in the bowl, not our typical mature, high-quality stocks. It was not a portfolio like any of our others, but it had our name on it and appeared in our quarterly report.

One day a former employee who'd gone to the city to seek his fortune called us up. "Is this John C. I'm reading about in the *New York Times* our John C.?"

"Huh?" I didn't know what he was talking about, so I went out and got the paper. Yes, you remember newspapers? You didn't yet just look online. I read the story, bug-eyed. It turns out that two adolescent boys in Westchester County had been found dead in a ditch, and as the investigation unfolded, detectives discovered there was a group of men in the county who had been making arrangements to meet young boys through an AOL chat room. They conducted a county-wide sweep to arrest these men, for "endangering the welfare of a minor," and possibly also for murder. *Our* John C. was captured in this net! I could tell because he was identified as a member of the school board.

Oh damn, damn, dammit ... our carefully cultivated reputation was suddenly in jeopardy! I'd never forgotten the venerated investor Warren Buffett's dictum: "It takes 20 years to build a reputation and five minutes to ruin it." It looked like this might be my five. Feeling a little sick inside, I called John C.'s house (landline, of course) to get more firsthand info and find out what was happening. There was no answer. I kept calling and calling. No answer. I called some more. Finally his teenage daughter picked up, and I asked for him. She said, in that sullen way of all teenagers, "He's out." I told her I really needed to speak to him. He was the only one who could make changes in his portfolio, and we were adrift without him. I kept talking and cajoling: "Where is he? This is urgent! ... When will he be back? ... It's totally important—when can I reach him? ... Do I have to drive down there now?"

Finally she broke, and said with an inflection that only a girl who'd spent time in public school and had learned to say multiple things at once could utter, "He's in trou-*bull*."

Uh-oh.

Yes, our guy was arrested as part of that major sweep, and he went to jail. Initially he got out on probation, but shortly thereafter a probation officer came snooping around his house and saw through the window that John had left out a VHS tape of *Le cage aux folles*. Dirty, really? But enough to violate his probation.

You can't make this stuff up. Nor can you make up the fact that he begged, within the six minutes allowed on a prison phone call, to continue to manage his strategy from jail, and described how he could do it. How his kids could visit and bring him the charts and data he needed. Indeed we actually thought for a minute about maybe letting that happen, since the alternative would have been to simply shut down the strategy with no cause given, which wouldn't look good on paper. Well, anyway, you can't have an employee or partner with a felony conviction in the highly regulated investment management business, so there wasn't in fact a choice. We had to wing it, managing the stocks ourselves until we could make a graceful exit and preserve our reputation. Meetings and more meetings and phone calls. Rationally it was, after all, a small part of our revenues, and probably not of existential impact. Still, there were late nights unable to get to sleep from the adrenaline rush generated by the absurdity of it all. ... *How could I wind up in this pickle? What can we say to our clients?*

It was a period of constant stress, as I lost control over the outcomes of my own efforts. I started to feel strange plaques on my scalp. Not mere dandruff, but the sort of bumps that would catch your fingertips as you stroked your hair. I recall I also started to burp a lot, which was peculiar, unfamiliar to me.

In January of 2002, I went downstairs in the morning to find that my legs were tingling from the knees down, tingling something like the feeling you get when your limbs "go to sleep," only I hadn't been in any kind of odd or stressed physical position. There was no cause that I knew of. Over the next few days, the tingling elided into more of a buzzing and grew stronger and stronger. It was mysterious. Soon enough the buzzing graduated into a burning, *burning* from my knees down to my feet, then quite quickly the burning sensation was focused on my feet, both feet at once. It was not mild. It was burning. I couldn't put on shoes. My life had become a kind of firewalk.

▪ ▪ ▪

I see now that my immune system had over time become a kind of metaphoric Popeye, as when that mumbling character said, *I can stands so much and I can't stands no more!* The mobilization of my natural immunity to suppress the persistent background growth of Borrelia began to come up short after 20 years in the face of the energetic upheavals produced by business anxiety and loss of control.

In a way it was the first moment of a longer-term breakdown, triggered by emotional shock. What seemed to be solid ground was solid no longer. Before this, I would get up every day and go to business work, or write, or train in aikido, and make sculpture in my studio. At night I would try to think about what it all means, and replay my day to observe how my brain functioned from scene to scene. It was a lovely modern-day Samuel Pepys existence. Each day, little wins and losses, and amusement at the whole of it.

But now I could barely get to sleep. My feet were burning me awake.

Finally, after so many years of tolerating depletion-induced fatigue, and bugs crawling under my skin (quite literally!), and an array of other symptoms that I considered minor and "just me" at the time (angry and unpredictable gut, overly sensitive sinuses, inexplicable heat in the head, frequent urination, persistent inflamed skin around my nose and chin), here was a really serious symptom—a five-alarm fire in my feet. Time to go into the medical system.

2002:
Doctor 1:
A First Mainstream Doctor

I still didn't have a regular doctor at the time (age 54, OMG), so I sought out an internist, believing that type was a more sophisticated all-around doctor than a simple GP. I found an internist with a decent vita (not so easy in my area), including undergrad at Brown, with a sweet little one-man office in an old stone building with creaky floors. His diplomas peppered the walls, and his demeanor was "kindly mature doctor giving full attention" with a sympathetic smile. I felt like a civilian, dwarfed by what must be his vast medical knowledge.

He suggested a test, as all doctors do. Ruling things in and ruling things out. Hoping to provide all the symptom information I could, I dropped my pants and showed him the persistent rashes on my inner thighs, which always appeared whenever I was tired or stressed. That didn't seem to register with him. I put my pants back on.

The test was some kind of machine that measures the electrical impulses of your nerves after stimulation, to see if there is any malfunction. There were many electrodes with wires hanging from those little white snap pads. The tech could tell me nothing, as they never do, but I soon had another appointment with my kindly-seeming internist shortly thereafter. In the meantime I began researching What Could This Pain in My Feet Possibly Be? There were more than 15 on the list, including diabetes, kidney disease, vitamin deficiency, hypothyroidism, injury, poisoning, hepatitis C, cancer, defective blood flow, and autoimmune diseases. I really had none of the additional symptoms that would point to a deeper look at any of these possibilities. I assumed blood tests would provide some further insight.

When we met for a discussion of my electromyography test, the doctor informed me, "Yes, you have a problem with the nerves in your legs, going down to your feet." I thought to myself, *Duh, that's why I came here.*

"So, what is it?" I said.

"We'll do some blood tests to rule out what we can." *OK*, I thought, *let's rule things out. Let's rule them out and throw them away.* I went from blood draw to blood draw, feet burning and burning. I kept reading, doing research, hoping for answers. Very few things can motivate one to swallow the dry taste of academic medical studies as vigorously as acute foot pain.

And so it came time to review the electromyography study alongside the blood tests. "Well," he said, "you clearly have a problem with the nerves in your legs, on both sides. But anyone looking at only your blood tests would say, 'There's a healthy 50-ish-year-old man.' We'll have to do some more tests."

Contemplating the prospect of a mystery ailment and pain lasting indefinitely only made my feet hurt even more. So I took out a sheaf of papers I'd printed up from my readings seeking answers; they filled the additional patient chair next to me.

"There's this fairly new thing going around in our area," I said, "called Lyme disease." I ran through some of the papers, a few of which were done by a doctor from Long Island (another hot spot, it turns out) named Burrascano, who'd basically devoted his life to Lyme research and left his private practice to do so. With my fingers unsteady from excitement over the possibility of an answer, I pointed out the section where he talked about rashes and fatigue and neuropathy as typical symptoms of Lyme infection after it had been present in the body for a while. Thinking that my internist and I were in it together to discover what was wrong with me, I said, "Looks like it could be Lyme. What do you think?"

The doctor asked me to gather up the papers and come into his office. He put on his kindest, most earnest and knowledgeable and sincere look, scrunching his eyebrows mid-forehead.

"Over the years," he said, "I've come to see there are just some situations with patients where we're not a good fit. So I think you need to find another doctor."

Holy shit! He fired me!

I should have known, and I certainly know by now, that doctors DO NOT want to get medical research information from their patients, no matter how credible the source. I can understand it in a way, because medicine and biology have disciplines and subtleties that the untrained can't grasp, and patients—in the eyes of their doctors—simply don't have access to the data from scientific studies that would change the picture and lead to different conclusions. Never mind that today on the internet anyone can access the latest information at credible sites like the NIH or *Frontiers in Medicine* or the CDC, or Mayo Clinic, or the various specialty associations of doctors and researchers. You'd think, given their busy schedules, that doctors would be interested in all the additional information they could get. After all, given the steady onrush of studies and developments, who has the time to keep up? Still, they don't want to waste their time, that precious time carved up into successive 22-minute profit opportunities each day.

Stay tuned. Later in the narrative this very doctor—Doctor 1—makes an almost Stendhalian appearance, as the plot unexpectedly turns back in his direction.

2002:
First Neurologist

Cast back out on the street, I took my nerve-test and blood results to an elderly neurologist, who wasn't so averse to the possibility of Lyme.

"Yes," he said, "it could be. Years ago when people came in with strange neurological symptoms, pretty much the last thing we did was test for Lyme. Now it's the first. I've got two guys in my practice down with it right now."

So he went through the first-visit neurological workup that was later to become all too familiar. The taps with the little hammer. The pricks with a needle. Do you feel that? The following of a finger with just my eyes. The forehead flicks. The walking along a straight line. All very serious.

In the end he said: "You might have Lyme. I'll order the test, but I have to tell you that the test isn't very accurate as far as we know. And even if it's positive, there's not much we can do about it."

He also ordered an EKG, since he'd already seen some cardio-system involvement from Lyme. Indeed, the test showed I had a right bundle branch block (RBBB in the medical profession). To be brief, running alongside the heart are bundles of "wires" conducting electricity that the "pump" can use; one bundle on the right and one on the left, a redundant system in which either side can do the job. Turns out RBBB is not that serious (my brother-in-law, a doctor, was born with it), but still, you're supposed to have two working bundles. I'd had physicals in the past, for sports or for insurance, and there had been no RBBB. In fact it's now known that *Borrelia* can infect and cause problems with the heart and vascular systems, including damaging the right bundle branch.

Feeling alone with these dissatisfying first encounters with mainstream doctors (even the good one said, "There's not much we can do about it"), I kept looking for answers. My feet continued to hurt. My mother lay dying in a hospital room. My feet hurt so badly I had to take off my shoes, and with some shame I sniffed that I hadn't washed my socks. I was in an animal panic to get rid of the pain. I had to find some way to fight the increased bouts of fatigue that had joined it by now as a stronger and debilitating symptom, attacking without warning.

2003:
Driven to the Alternatives

A few people told me about a doctor an hour away who'd developed a practice specializing in Lyme. Supposedly he'd already treated some 5,000 Lyme cases, which is a lot considering how few doctors had even heard of the disease then. Having decided by then that my best shot at a diagnosis was Lyme—I could find no other condition that fit—I pointed myself in his direction. Turned out he was what was then called an "alternative" or "complementary" doctor, an MD who'd use whatever he thought might work, no matter what the Infectious Diseases Society of America (IDSA) had to say.

Today those alt docs practice what's called "functional medicine," but it's still the same rather woo-woo approach. Here you'll find everything from Rife machines (which produce magnetic pulses) to hyperthermic cures (high heat), to hypothermic approaches (temporary freezing, basically), to burning candles in the ears to "withdraw toxins," to controlled bee stings, to lasers, to complete blood exchanges. I encountered this sort of practitioner when a friend's wife had stage IV lung cancer and he was convinced to lug her all the way to Germany so her blood could be purified of the glucose that allegedly fed the cancer—all for a tidy sum.

An article from the early 2000s (though it could really have been relevant at any point in human history) published by the NIH states the following:

> For these devices or methods, no proper clinical trials are done or discussed. No phase I trials to assess toxicity, no phase II trials to assess efficacy and no phase III trials to compare with standard therapies. There is no ethics committee approval and patients are not asked to sign a consent form stating that they are enrolled in a trial of an investigational therapy. However, they may be asked to sign a waiver to "cover" the person treating them, acknowledging that the therapy is not accepted by the medical establishment. This, they are assured, does not mean that the treatment does not work, "it is just a legal requirement to satisfy the regulators." The practitioner may adopt the wry smile of an embattled innovator struggling with the uncaring forces of government regulation. The therapist may claim to be conducting research, but there is no ethics approval and the results of well-conducted clinical trials are not published in respected journals.
>
> Advertising emphasizes anecdotes and testimonials but never quotes the most relevant type of research: the controlled clinical trial. However, unlike many other types of al-

> ternative medicine, the claims for these medical devices are dressed up with plausible-sounding bits of scientific jargon. The therapist may say that this treatment will "help the immune system fight cancer" or that it will "starve the cancer of the glucose it needs to survive." The therapist may use a device that will "scan your body" or "analyze" your blood or a hair sample and detect critical nutritional deficiencies or imbalances that you need to correct to survive your cancer. The therapist will claim to have special knowledge that is not accepted by the established medical profession.
> (https://www.ncbi.nlm.nih.gov/pmc/articles/PMC3097732/)

Never mind, my feet were like sirens driving me for relief. So far, conventional science had nothing to offer. Like many patients who show up for functional treatment after conventional medicine failures, or who just don't "believe" in what the white coats are saying, I was desperate. I didn't know it at the time, but plenty more desperation lay in wait.

I found the driveway for the New Era Deep Healing Center on a rainy afternoon in September. This new doctor was yet another internist, but one who'd left the fold for "alternative" approaches. I was ready with an envelope of cash, which I was told to bring because the doctor didn't take insurance and required an "initial consultation fee" that was about five times what one would expect to pay a conventional doctor for a consultation.

> Then there is the money. No matter how simple the treatment seems, it will be expensive. It may seem tailored to the amount that the person seems likely to be able to afford. Special discounts may be offered to those with less money, or a cheaper "but just as effective" form of the therapy may unexpectedly become available for those with financial prob-

> lems. Often treatment with the unproven medical device is just one of a menu of treatments available at an alternative cancer treatment center. One may also find homeopathy, iridology, naturopathy, orthomolecular medicine and other mutually contradictory members of the complementary and alternative medicine family available.

OK, I had the money. Honestly, if they'd told me I'd have to give them *all* my money to get relief from the pain, I would have at least considered it.

I went into the waiting room and found a somewhat unexpected wall of racks filled with marketing materials and order forms for various vitamins and supplements. They were from suppliers in California and Argentina and Canada, companies with no logos but just block letters announcing their names at the top of ordinary printer paper. Did I need the purest B12? Bee pollen from Nova Scotia? Elixir of mint made with special spring water that had been controlled by the Iroquois for hundreds of years? A mushroom mix that would get rid of the heavy metals in my blood and kill anaplasma bacteria at the same time?!

My father had a law practice in a very conservative, waspy town, and he was also a professor at a prestigious law school in New York City. We had conversations about professional responsibility and ethics at the dinner table. Notions about conflict of interest occupied many cubbies in my brain. So my dismay at seeing these supplement order forms doubled when I noticed that at the bottom of the forms was the doctor's name stamped in red ink. Oh, I saw, he was due to get credit, and presumably a commission, on each one. Oh boo. Creepy. But never mind—just then, my feet were roused up and on fire. I was hardly ready to ditch this project over my concerns as to the dubious ethics of running a practice where you sell what you prescribe. I gave it a pass, my need for relief overruling my moralizing reactions.

The doc had a nice and genial manner. He was a steady smiler, eyebrows high and rounded, with his own version of the confident, knowledgeable professional demeanor that MDs master. This version leaned more friendly than stern, buttressed by a pose of sympathy and concern. He had the air of a warrior in the battle against Lyme, an explorer enjoying his time in the wild. He was going to win against *Borrelia*! He could feel it, and I could feel him feeling it.

I recapped my history, including the massive summer flu 20 years earlier. When I was finished, he said, "We'll do the Western blot test." At this time the Western blot wasn't as common in testing for Lyme as it is now, so he was ahead of the game here. "But I'm quite sure you have Lyme. The clinical history is easily just as important as any test, especially because the diagnostics aren't perfect. When the clinical history and symptoms say Lyme, the test almost always agrees."

So then he gave me a box from a lab in California with a name like "LabX," also with his name stamped in red on the bottom. "You have to go to this lab. None of the regular commercial labs are able to do the test correctly. I'll draw some blood here, and we'll send it out overnight." His tone was intimate, as though he was just sharing this secret with me confidentially, as though he hadn't said it 5,000 times before. I sat there listening like a rube, with my lower lip hanging down, nodding in assent.

OK, that's my introduction to a functional medicine doctor. Apparently once you have your MD degree and state license, you can go and do *whatever*. To shorten this segment, I'll note that my guy explained that this *Borrelia* bacteria was a nasty little sucker and we'd have to go right into antibiotics. ("It can put on a cloak and hide from the immune system," he explained, a kind of cartoon version of something we know today to be correct.)

Once the test result came from LabX and read positive for Lyme, he began prescribing one antibiotic after another. Their names blurred into each other. He created antibiotic cocktails. He gave me something called Mepron, which is a malaria medicine, just in case I also had babesiosis, a coinfection that also comes from the *Ixodes* bite. That stuff really made me nauseated, and I was ready to get well immediately if I didn't have to take it anymore. We went through doxycycline, amoxicillin, ampicillin, all the -cillins, tetracycline, other -ines. I can't even remember them all. There were usually at least two different pills at once. This went on, trial and error, for about a year. I was rattled; months and months at a time on antibiotics, one after another. But he told me that was necessary. "We have to try things to see what works for each individual," he explained.

My gut did not thank me, and I began to take up bathroom reading. Even started on some ideas for a product called "Toilet Table" that you could flip up to hold your books or magazines nicely while you dealt with the side effects of all these antibiotics, which kill the good bacteria in your intestines along with everything else. Note that up to 3% of cells by weight in the body are composed of microorganisms, and by number there are 10 trillion. When you're sending in the troops against *Borrelia*, there is bound to be some collateral microbial damage.

Unfortunately, this heaving of antibiotics against my infection (essentially like tossing antibiotic spaghetti against a bacterial wall to see what will stick) did not really add up to much symptom relief. The state of proven treatment was not very different than it had been 20 years prior for my friend Howard, who was an even earlier adopter of Lyme than I. Burning foot pain and fatigue still ruled my day.

2003:
I Meet Ketek

But I noted in one appointment with my woo-doc that Joseph Burrascano (my guy was a follower of his) had changed his protocol to include a drug called telithromycin (trade name Ketek) in his most recent update on Lyme treatment—Burrascano had a kind of white paper that he updated every two or three years. I asked about it, because in the paper he said Ketek was the best performer against Lyme and was his personal choice. I'd never heard of it before. It's an interesting drug because it is bacteri*cidal,* whereas most antibiotics are bacterio*static*—meaning that the latter simply slow down the bacteria's growth (hence *-static*), in hopes that the natural immune system can finish the job, whereas bactericidal drugs actually kill (*-cidal*) what they find.

Do they kill it all? Well, at that time there wasn't a good way to know, and even today, almost 25 years after my first visit with this alternative doc, Lyme diagnostic science hasn't advanced far enough to know any more than that the body had a *Borrelia* infection sometime in the past. That leaves a footprint, which unfortunately interferes with identifying a current infection. There is a way to tell if there's a recent bite (IgM bands showing on the Western blot) or if there's been one in the past (IgG bands on the blot), but *no* real quantitative way to tell whether a treatment has reduced the level of infection today (!!!!&*&^%$#^!!!!). If you should happen to find some cells in a blood draw, that would be a coincidence. Science is left with only inferential evidence of infection—the continued presence of antibodies. How much information is that? Well, for example, almost everyone has evidence of antibodies to past Epstein-Barr virus (EBV, notably implicated in mononucleosis) infection in their blood. But hardly anyone actually *has* current Epstein-Barr illness.

Anyway, since my guy was apart from the insurance system, I managed to get my newly acquired GP—illness had made me all grown up, with a regular doctor—to write me a covered script. She lit up. "Oh yes, that's a wonderful drug," she said, almost starry-eyed. That was reassuring, since she'd been trained in the navy and there was nothing alternative about her. Anyway, damned if that Ketek didn't begin to induce some improvement within the first month. Yay! Still, my feet burned and I fell asleep in any silent pause. The symptoms were, however, much less severe than before, and I could sleep at night because the burning had let up just enough to let me enter the deep respite of slumber. After many months and many combinations of antibiotics that failed, Ketek gave clear signs that it might work. And, interestingly, not only was Ketek gut-sparing, but during the successive six-week periods when I was dosing with it, my gut behaved better than I could ever remember in my adult life.

The next 10 to 15 years were, with one major interruption, my Golden Age of Ketek. That drug gave me my life back.

I resumed the multivariate, high-energy world that had filled my younger self. During these years I collected many of the badges of society—though accumulating credits was never my conscious project. (I see this only in retrospect; the markers were merely the consequence or result of following my nose to what gave me joy, enthusiasm, or the feeling of expansiveness.)

My business grew to notable size. I and we had plenty of media placements (*Wall Street Journal,* Bloomberg, CNBC, Barron's, etc.), and a kind of fame among advisors and their clients seeking an investment edge. I published a book on dividend stock investing that was soon cited on many "best investment books" lists. Our firm became the largest employer in town. People who worked for us bought houses, had children, and joined many of the local charities and arts organizations the business regularly supported. My sculpture started being selected for regional and national group shows by curators with major reputations in the art world. Meanwhile, a popular reference book I had produced became an annual selection of the Book of the Month Club (yes, that was back in the day) and sold many hundreds of thousands of copies in various editions. A high-energy life that would make any mother proud, right?

But every six months or so, the wheels would start to slow down. I'd be sitting at my desk and feel my eyes begin to close, and close again when I tried to open them. Everything made me sad. All I wanted to do was sleep. So I'd get a new prescription for my friend Ketek and be fine, and resume my normal self again, lively for the next half year. Back to a full life, a happy feeling all day long, even for no reason. That telithromycin saw me through the early aughts and the teens, working with my immune system, I see in retrospect, to suppress the muck of slow-growing *Borrelia* in my body. It did a great job. I was surprised I didn't hear more about it in the Lyme readings I regularly perused. Though it was produced by a Big Pharma company as a treatment for bacterial pneumonia, doctors didn't seem to be aware that it was potent against *Borrelia*.

It did a great job compared with everything else, but not a perfect job.

2012:
Monster Face

One day in 2012, I was driving home from an aikido class on the short country back road that led to my home. That road is lined with trees, often second or third growth, and if the sun is bright and at the right angle, it creates a kind of blinding stroboscopic effect, flashing in between the tree trunks as you drive along. It makes you slow down. But this day the strobe effect was different. It was stronger, and was a faster vibration than merely the flashes of sun I was used to. My vision got a little blurry too. What was going on? Would I be able to make it home OK? Mercifully the road was only a couple of miles long, and I pulled into my driveway just fine. I told my wife about it, changed, showered, and eased into bed.

The next morning my wife was horrified. My face was twisted, my mouth drooping on the left side, and my left eye would not open. She hustled me into the car and drove me to the hospital ER a couple of towns over. We said nothing on the way; it seemed a serious moment when whatever had gone wrong just might be major. We didn't want to speculate. I just put my seat back and closed my eyes. The daylight was hurting them, making them ache.

In the hospital a female Russian doctor examined me. She put out her hands and counted off my symptom display finger by finger, going through the eyes, the mouth, the sensitivities, one by one as if marching down the list of a med school textbook she'd memorized. She paused and contemplated what she'd just adumbrated.

"It's not a stroke," she said. "It's Bell's palsy." She listed what we were going to do about it, including antibiotics and the steroid prednisone, and opined that it was not life-threatening and would go away with her prescribed treatment and plenty of rest. She gave me a black patch to cover my left eye, which had begun to ooze pus, and gave my wife a treatment protocol.

Bell's palsy! (Paralysis of the seventh cranial nerve, which controls tiny muscles and nerves around the eyes and lips.) This I already knew to be a standard Lyme symptom. My friend Howard already had it. It's prominent on the symptom list for Lyme, so typical that it could almost serve as a diagnostic touchstone. But most often it occurs early in the disease, within the first year or so, as when Howard had gotten it. My Bell's was really late, rising up like some geological event that had been suppressed by the heavy rocks above for years until it burst through.

This put me in bed with my door shut. I holed up with my computer and didn't go into the office for nearly six months, telling my employees they'd just have to carry on without me. My face was monstrous, with an ugly sneer permanently plastered on it. I couldn't go outside because the daylight literally hurt my eyes, as though someone were punching the eyeballs. I learned why we are born with eyelids: when you can't fully close your eyelids, the shampoo will go right in there and sting like hell.

I managed to get out of the house for a trip back to the neurologist I'd seen back in 2002, the one who was decently aware of Lyme, unlike so many doctors even at that time, 25 years after the discovery of it. He gave me the full workup again, with the little hammers, the pinpricks, the tuning forks, the mild laser beam for me to follow. He got close to my face, looked deeply into my eyes, and said, "It's Bell's palsy, and I think it's from Lyme." I noted he was a shade less than definitive. He didn't or couldn't say just plain "It's from Lyme." Why? There was still no test to show for sure that a Lyme case was a Lyme case and no other thing.

To rule out other causes, he set me up for an MRI of my head and neck. Things were pretty normal, but the radiologist's comment, unprompted, was that he observed "punctate white matter intensities and inflammation typical of Lyme disease." They can't actually see a specific infection in the brain happening, but in magnetic resonance images they can see the trail of reaction or damage that it leaves.

Ulp. The buggers were in my brain!

What a strange feeling, to know a parasite is inhabiting or has inhabited one's own brain. What to do about it? I'm an American man, so of course my first thought was to *do something* and fix the problem. But that would have to wait. The first order was learning to live at least transiently with a twisted face, an eye that wouldn't close, and photophobia, or vision that was intensely reactive to light, especially to daylight.

The neurologist explained that most cases of Bell's palsy "resolve" in 6 to 12 months, meaning that the nerves heal over time without external treatment. But, he said, in a phrase I had come to hear too many times, "yours is a bad one." Mercifully I could do my work from home—especially important because this was just at a time when my business was gathering momentum, reaching 65 employees and multiple billions under management. Despite all this, I couldn't go in to meet with the team, in part because I didn't want folks to see me looking like the lead in a monster movie, and in part because my lips wouldn't work correctly. I recall noting that I couldn't say "fuck" (though of course I wanted to all the time), but I could easily say "puck." Interesting insight on the facial muscle involvement in elocution ... Too, I couldn't keep both eyes open without the bad one watering and producing a little rivulet down my cheek. As you can imagine, my body was beaten up over this, craving sleep and rest as much as possible, though that was a conflict with my generally forward-charging nature.

One day I noticed that the smell of my armpits had changed. Researching this, I found that the facial nerves—which basically short-circuit and blow like overcharged wires during Bell's palsy—heal by first dissolving, basically rotting, into the body, before regrowing again like green shoots after a forest fire. That smell was the smell of dying nerves, dead nerves dissolving and dissipating in one of the incredible homeostatic maneuvers of the magical human multivariate system.

Still, sometimes duty calls, and I doubt I'll soon forget a manager due diligence meeting with Citicorp in New York City. Getting in front of the approvers so my firm could be authorized for use by their advisors had been a multiyear process, and it just didn't seem we could pass up the opportunity for a meeting when it arose. So our marketing people packed me up in the back seat of my car, put pillows under my head and over my eyes, and drove to New York City, about two hours south, on a painfully sunny weekday afternoon. I wanted to vomit most of the way, but somehow kept it down. When we arrived, they held my arm for support as I hobbled from the parking garage, darkest of dark sunglasses perched on my nose over a black eye patch. *This is ridiculous*, I thought. *How will I ever talk to them? How will they ever want to hire a firm whose founder and president is scary and unbearable to look at?* The Citicorp people were young, though, and they must have taken pity on this older guy with a profound issue; by some miracle we passed the review to approval. Could my condition have been relatable? I wouldn't have thought so, but perhaps young bureaucrats don't have the instinctive, visceral human reactions I surely would have had. I would have said let's wait and see this guy again when he's better—*if* he's ever going to be whole again.

Actually, thanks to Ketek, over time he did get better, if not exactly whole. Bit by bit, the movement came back into my face over the next year. I could drink juice from a glass without getting half the liquid on my shirt. Then I learned to press hard and suck it up through a straw. I learned to wash my hair without letting the soap go anywhere near my non-closing left eye. By and by, I learned to force that eye shut for a few precious seconds while I lathered my head. I learned to eat on the right side of my mouth, as it wouldn't open large enough to get a fork in on the left. It took half a year before I could go outside without feeling like someone was hitting my eyes with a hard stick, but I could read again, covering up the bad eye with one hand. That stranger's face is still distorted, even to this day, though more mildly, and the photophobia is still present, though, again, mildly. Foot burning was replaced by the sensation of walking on stones. At times I bent over to scrape off what was on my sole and irritating me like a stone or a safety pin, but found nothing there.

Oh geez, I thought, *all of it produced by a tiny, tiny tick, with an even tinier microbe inside it, from a time when nobody knew their names.*

A FEW THINGS ABOUT LYME

But fatigue and Bell's palsy are not death, eye pain is not blindness, foot burning is not amputation. One can still touch, and hear, just as before; the symptoms are debilitating but not existential or mortal—and that's why, it seems to me, so little has been done by the medical/research establishment in terms of accurate diagnosis and therapeutic treatment or cure since the first Connecticut reports of disease clusters arose in 1976.

Indeed, you can have the disease without symptoms—I've seen many anecdotal reports of symptom-free infections for 10 years or more (I am one of them)—depending on how your immune system handles invaders. So one factor is the character of your immune system, and the other is that *Borrelia burgdorferi* is well known to be a slow grower, finding suitable habitats inside the body where it can live long, feeding entirely on LDH (lactate dehydrogenase, a by-product of the breakdown of glucose in the body—to be discussed later) and quite content to simply replicate, until your immune system hits a moment of maximum accretion, becoming angry and inflamed over the presence of fully recognized alien life inside where it doesn't belong.

According to clinical studies (and even autopsies, ugh) *Borrelia* can live, and rather enjoys living, in many amenable spots across the corporeal landscape. One of the most common destinations is in the joints, as in the case of my friend Howard. One often hears about this, especially in relatively new cases, and it even has a name: Lyme arthritis. This is painful and feels like acute arthritis, though it's not actual arthritis, which involves degradation of joint cartilage, often brought about by wear and tear or growth of bone in the wrong place, producing pain and stiffness in hands, ankles, knees, hips, and spine—all the joints that move. In both instances the body's response is inflammation. In arthritis it is from physical rubbing or friction or nerve impingement, while in Lyme the symptoms come from an immune response targeting *Borrelia* where it doesn't belong, something like the way an oyster targets a grain of sand, neutralizing it with pearl. There are Lyme arthritis cases that include partial or full paralysis, although, as I've come to see, that paralysis could be a result of *Borrelia* infection of the spinal cord and/or its meningeal sheath.

Clearly, Lyme can find its way into the central nervous system; it demonstrably likes to live on or near nerves, accounting for Bell's palsy, pain, weakness, numbness, meningitis, visual disturbances, and other neurological symptoms. These are very similar to the symptoms of multiple sclerosis (MS), and in the literature there are numerous cases of patients who remained untreated for Lyme while their physicians remained incorrectly convinced they had MS. Lupus is another misdiagnosis, as are chronic fatigue syndrome, fibromyalgia, Epstein-Barr, cellulitis, migraine, and so on. Thus Lyme has become known as the Great Imitator, or the Great Impostor. Symptoms can present in such a way as to lead doctors in the wrong direction. But since I'm not a doctor, I can tell you what the *right* direction is: all infection symptoms are caused by an inflammatory response by the immune system. It's not the microbe or anything it emits. (I can recall in the early days when both conventional and complementary practitioners would say the *Borrelia* "gave off a toxin." They might as well have been talking about "vapors.") Even COVID, when it becomes long-haul, has a similar symptom set to that of Lyme. That's because the immune response is similar, although COVID is a virus and Lyme is a bacteria.

Symptoms don't emit from an infection, but ensue from the body's attempt to heal it. Too much immune activity becomes self-defeating, as when persistent vomiting up of toxins winds up causing dehydration and systemic collapse. As researcher Michal Caspi Tal of MIT has noted, "the immune system can kill you." We'll talk more about that apparent paradox later on. In the meantime, it's important to note why Lyme has remained enigmatic to the medical community, and why the disease is so difficult to diagnose directly (as opposed to simply identifying antibodies).

Many illnesses have an active agent that can be seen under a microscope, or in medical imaging. In the case of microbes, they are cultured outside the body to find an antibiotic or antifungal that's likely to kill or retard them. In the case of Lyme, however, as Ying Zhang of Johns Hopkins put it, "*Borrelia* doesn't culture." It might be possible to capture an individual microbe from a blood draw and determine its DNA, but the odds against that would be so great as to make it random. It would be like panning for biological gold in a place where no other gold has been found, and it would not be useful for diagnostics.

Back to the story.

Over the next years I regained most of my past state, regained some measure of health and energy. I could go out, with my face only moderately disfigured, no longer prompting children to ask what was the matter with my mouth. I had what everyone wants, which is the feeling of making *progress* in life. My business continued to grow exponentially, gaining new customers who sought something "real" after the devastation of the 2008–9 financial crises. My sculpture was gaining a following on Instagram and in juried shows. My family flourished, everyone making progress, progress. By fall of 2014, I married the wonderful woman I'd lived with for 20 years in a rather epic wedding. Also that summer I'd had a one-man show in Woodstock that was well received—at the end I didn't feel there was anything more I could have done for it, didn't feel like I'd missed any chances; I was content with what I'd done (a pretty rare feeling for me). My firm had managed to get some publicly traded products off the ground, and I rang the opening bell at the New York Stock Exchange three times in 2014–15.

These badges are what we seek to feel potent, and to provide the illusion that time and effort are cumulative, building toward something bigger and better. They formed a constellation of little wins that diverted my attention, that helped me ignore the festering bacteria that would knock me down as if on cue every six months or so, putting me on my back into a plunging depression and fatigue. Then I would, as I had for over 10 years since meeting up with Woo-Doc, dose up with Ketek and jog on to the next relapse and downfall, feeling pretty much fine until it happened. I knew, if perhaps not with the kind of certainty that an opiate addict might have, that I was dependent on the drug. I knew, in the way you hear a small voice inside but do anything you can to avoid hearing it, life would go downhill without my dear telithromycin.

KETEK HAS A STORY OF ITS OWN

But all was not well on the Ketek front. Like our small-cap manager John C., Ketek, it turns out, was in trou-*bull*. There was plenty of evidence that it elevated liver enzymes. That in itself is not so bad, or even unusual for effective drugs. But before too long there were reports from Europe—where it had been approved in 2001, a few years before the US approval—of actual liver injury. As I understand it, most of those reports had to do with children taking the drug, and the fact is that overall there were only some 35 reports from among the more than 5 million patients who'd used it.

For context, telithromycin was originally approved as a treatment for bacterial community-acquired pneumonia (CAP), and as such, was seen to be by far the most effective drug against CAP, which is often fatal. (I think most of the elderly people I've known who've passed have died of pneumonia, acquired in the hospital as often as not. It's far deadlier than COVID, for example). Recall that Ketek works so well because it is bactericidal; it kills the bacteria, rather than simply slowing down bacterial growth (that is, acting bacteriostatically), as do most antibiotics.

But here the plot thickened. It was discovered that in the original submission to the FDA, one of the researchers, Maria Anne Kirkman Campbell, had fabricated her data. She went to prison for 57 months for the fraudulent reporting (the charges included mail fraud), though her portion of the original study was 400 patients out of 24,000 (in study number 3014). This failure of proper research protocols in combination with reports of discrete liver injury (though they were rare compared with the number of users) prompted the FDA to issue a "black box" warning on the drug, limiting it to fewer indications and strongly prohibiting its use in cases of myasthenia gravis (MG), which is a disease in which the communication between nerves and muscles breaks down, cursing the patient to basically lose control of their body in a kind of Gumby collapse.

A terrible thing, to be sure, but it does raise the question of how an antibiotic might exacerbate an autoimmune disease that is not bacterial in origin. My AI tells me that MG is genetic in origin or due to a faulty thymus gland. The body is filled with wonders and mysteries; since I'm not a doctor, I'll just have to accept that through some inexplicable process an antibiotic can have a strong impact on what is apparently not a bacterial infection. Scientists may well have an answer. This complex body ...

Lo! some further research suggests that other antibiotics in specific classes, such as ciprofloxacin (Cipro) and levofloxacin (Levaquin)—our friends against anthrax—azithromycin, and erythromycin, can also interfere with neuromuscular transmission. They also pose an apparent, if small, danger to the liver.

But this association with myasthenia gravis does prompt still more questions: Why are these latter drugs still on the market? Why was Ketek first black boxed, then for all practical purposes banned, even though it is the best performer against both Lyme and the often-fatal community-acquired pneumonia?

We're in the realm of conspiracy theories here, but I suggest that Aventis (the company marketing Ketek then) profoundly annoyed and angered the FDA staff by presenting data that was in part fraudulent (though in fact it was a small section of the total study backing up the application for approval, and didn't actually undermine the vast majority of the data). The collective faces of the researchers and scientists wound up spattered with egg—the egg of shame and the egg of anger. Medical scientists and government bureaucrats can't tolerate mistakes in data, much less deception. Nor do they appreciate getting snookered in their decision-making. (The fraud wasn't discovered until after Ketek received formal approval.) Plus, there is the legal exposure that could develop from approval of an improperly tested and presented drug. The professional ignominy of having to essentially retract an approval that had already been given is a wound that won't heal quickly.

Lots of things can insult the liver, including regular wine with meals. Indeed, Morgan Spurlock's documentary film Super Size Me demonstrated the liver insult that can be generated by merely eating nothing but McDonald's for 30 days. Indeed, at the end of the adventure his liver enzymes were elevated, perhaps similar to what might be seen in the cited Ketek cases. But McDonald's never submitted partially false data to the FDA, so they're still around. Just sayin'. ...

But wait, there's more.

There must have been a large inventory of Ketek in the system, because I had no trouble picking it up at my local chain pharmacy for a few years after the drug's manufacture was terminated in 2016.

But the day came when the pharmacy told me, "We don't carry that anymore." Picture my very sad face as an emoji with drooping lips; how would I procure Ketek to keep my Lyme under control? It turns out I'd been living off the remaining inventory scraps without knowing it. However, at my firm we had some international business, and the guy in charge of that explained to me he could still get Ketek in France (what's now Sanofi-Aventis is a Swiss company), and once or twice a year on his return trips he'd sneak in an envelope full of those pale orange pills to keep me going.

I knew I was on borrowed time, but I was excited to see that a new drug, solithromycin, from the new, small company Cempra, had applied for FDA approval in 2015. It was targeted to CAP and proved superior to the standard CAP treatments of levofloxacin and ciprofloxacin, with far fewer side effects. Of course no one was testing it for Lyme, but what excited me was that solithromycin was actually telithromycin version 2.0! It was a much more effective bactericidal version of Ketek, with—and now I'm above my pay grade—three touch points on the bacteria, instead of two for other macrolides. The early tests against pneumonia proved overwhelmingly positive, and without the negative side effects—just some minor elevation of liver enzymes, not actual damage, nothing to see here. Those previous threats to the liver were caused by something that had been corrected in solithromycin. Imagine my joy at the new prospective availability of a safe antibiotic even more effective than Ketek. Yay!

All the arrows pointed to a drug as effective as Ketek, perhaps more so, without the harmful liver effects. I followed the news of soli's development carefully. The timeline had gone like this for the new drug, which Cempra had presented to the FDA:

- May 2011: Solithromycin is in a Phase 2 clinical trial for serious community-acquired bacterial pneumonia and in a Phase 1 clinical trial with an intravenous formulation.

- September 2011: Solithromycin demonstrated comparable efficacy to levofloxacin with reduced adverse events in Phase 2 trial in people with community-acquired pneumonia.
- January 2015: In a Phase 3 clinical trial for community-acquired bacterial pneumonia, solithromycin administered orally demonstrated statistical non-inferiority to the fluoroquinolone moxifloxacin.
- July 2015: Patient enrollment for the second Phase 3 clinical trial (Solitaire IV) for community-acquired bacterial pneumonia was completed with results expected in Q4 2015.
- October 2015: IV to oral solithromycin demonstrated statistical non-inferiority to IV to oral moxifloxacin in adults with community-acquired bacterial pneumonia.
- July 2016: Cempra announced FDA acceptance of IV and oral formulations of Solithera (solithromycin) new drug application for the treatment of community-acquired bacterial pneumonia.

You could feel the weather changing. The data was presented, and the advisory committee of the FDA (they review drugs before there's a full decision) had nothing but wonderful things to say about the drug's efficacy. (Drugs are viewed in terms of efficacy and safety.) Indeed, the committee voted 12–0 positive regarding efficacy, a unanimity rarely seen. In other words, the drug was potent. It really worked.

But there was history here, institutional history, and that dried egg to clean up. For it turns out Cempra's lead scientist (and president at the time) was the very same woman who had, some 12 years earlier, led the submission of Ketek, complete with its partly fraudulent data. This is why solithromycin appeared to be the new and improved telithromycin (Ketek). The same person had developed both!

Oh snap. Suspenseful music. One could imagine that the moment of revenge for her earlier humiliation of the FDA was at hand. So yes, they agreed the drug was effective. But they then followed that statement with this: "Some patients presented with elevated liver enzymes which may or may not be indicative of hepatotoxicity." This prompted the FDA Antimicrobial Drugs Advisory Committee to add, in sublimely bureaucratic language, that "risk to the liver has not been adequately characterized" and that further studies needed to be conducted. For this reason, the FDA requested a 9,000-patient safety trial.

Bear in mind that to demand of a small company like Cempra a 9,000-patient study (which would need to be made up of patients with current CAP who were willing to be part of a double-blind study), a study that would require tens or even hundreds of millions of dollars and perhaps two or more years, is essentially to refuse approval without actually formally rejecting it. Basically, they told the researcher/promoter, "Nice work, here's a gut punch for you."

Shortly thereafter she retired, or was retired, from Cempra, and nothing substantive has been heard of solithromycin ever since. And it won't be, unless there is a major health crisis and only solithromycin can resolve it.

With the palace intrigue over, I was left with no resort to deal with my persistent population of *Borrelia* and the immune system responses it provoked. My GP suggested trying amoxicillin again as a replacement for Ketek, only it turned out that members of the penicillin family are notorious for prompting antibiotic-associated diarrhea (post-antibiotic syndrome), and about a month after I finished a four-week course (which had no effect on my Lyme symptoms), I embarked on a continuous year of diarrhea, and an extended process of discovering the value of psyllium husk as a binder. Let's say it all made travel rather difficult. Not exactly a Lyme symptom, but part of the process.

So we're up to 2017. My life is burdened by unrelieved bouts of fatigue and bounded by a cap on energy output that, if exceeded, will result in a kind of collapse. My feet still burn (especially if the market is volatile! Stress matters!), and my vision is still hypersensitive to light, but it is nevertheless possible to push through in life. In addition, after all, I'm getting older, nearly 70 now. Am I feeling age, as much as Lyme?

2017:
Down the Research Rabbit Hole

In any event, because there were no newly developed drugs for Lyme since I'd started Ketek, it didn't seem as though mainstream medicine would have much to offer me. Merely looking in the mirror and catching sight of my still-disfigured face gave me the message that I should be looking into all the newest research, or seeking a different path, lest this festering colony of bacteria within rouse up another unexpected headline symptom. When I was depleted, the sensation of bugs crawling under the skin of my arms was another reminder that all was not well below the surface.

At this point, the quest for more and better doctors was not urgent. Let's face it, you can't go to a new doctor and tell her, "I've had bugs crawling under the skin of my arms ever since I had a severe flu in August, 35 years ago." You're just not going to get a lot of action on that. Or you'll get the wrong kind.

With a background doing critical analysis as an investment manager, and now with internet access exposing an almost unthinkable depth of credible information, I pumped up my earlier hobby: extensive medical research. I gathered up data—literally from around the globe, as Lyme disease was becoming increasingly common in Germany, Scandinavia, France, Central Europe, and East Asia. I was at all the government sites worldwide. You'd see me in the specialists' societies/associations' search boxes. My dog-ears were on the medical journals. I was in the back of the room at important specialty conferences.

Sorry to say there was little new to be found in terms of treatment for Lyme, especially for long-term Lyme, some 40 years after the disease had first been identified. Perhaps things have moved an inch: before 2010 it was the default position of the IDSA (Infectious Diseases Society of America) that "most Lyme infections can be cured with a relatively short term treatment of doxycycline." The CDC parroted this position in its treatment guidelines. And that may still be true. When the bite is recent and *Borrelia* spirochetes are still circulating in the blood, they are fairly susceptible to doxycycline treatment, and the body's immune system can be additionally effective against them, generating, among other immunity tools, fevers that are fatal to the bacteria. However, until 2010 the IDSA, again parroted by the CDC, took the position that there was no such thing as chronic Lyme, or late-stage Lyme, or long-term Lyme, call it what you will. In effect, any persistent symptoms were in the mind of the patient. This gaslighting from the "official" sources for Lyme "knowledge" resulted in untold suffering among hundreds of thousands of patients, and multiple misdiagnoses leading to further ineffective treatments. Since medical science could not "locate" Lyme in the body with any precision, the consequent conclusion was that persistent Lyme symptoms did not exist. It must be something other than Lyme, was the claim.

But by roughly 2010, the numbers of Lyme patients and long-term complaints had grown to a point where they could no longer be ignored, and additional study of the patient population led by Dr. John Aucott of Johns Hopkins concluded that yes, many patients who had not been treated in the early stages, in addition to as many as 20% of *treated* patients, developed a shared set of symptoms that lasted for months and could last, as the CDC put it, "for years." A new term entered the medical establishment, coined, I believe, by Dr. Aucott: *post-treatment Lyme disease syndrome*, or PTLDS. The IDSA and its followers, including the CDC, could buttress the dam of ignorance no longer. It had been pierced not by some bearded shaman outsider, but by one of their own.

Doctors were guided from that point to agree that maybe the patient-reported debilitation wasn't psychosomatic after all but could be real ... at least 20% of the time (!). There was still no data on a 40-year-old case like mine, but at least I could hold my head up high when explaining to some new doctor that I had PTLDS. Kind of amazing that giving it a name suddenly made it real. And I could say to myself, *Darn it, I've had post-treatment Lyme disease syndrome all these years. The fatigue, the burning feet, the Bell's palsy, the right bundle branch block. All post-treatment Lyme. PTLDS!*

I was sure that new research was on the way that would clear me up. Every month, it seemed, there was some new breakthrough in the labs that pointed the way to treatment, or at least to the behavior and life cycle of *Borrelia*, that would lead to a cure before long. Various university professors announced lab discoveries of new antibiotics. From a university near Boston came word of the discovery that an older antibiotic, hygromycin A, which had been mostly abandoned in earlier years because it was ineffective against most pathogens, turned out to be somehow *selectively targeted to Borrelia*, and killed it quickly. Plus, because it was kind of feeble regarding other kinds of bacteria, it was gut-sparing—it didn't disturb the GI system and cause diarrhea as did all the existing broad-spectrum antibiotics. Miracles and wonder!

As I did further digging, I noticed that the scientist who'd discovered, or rediscovered, hygromycin A had started a company to, a press release proclaimed, "develop and commercialize the opportunity." That phrase clanged in my skull. Is our capitalist system really a beautiful manifestation of the ability of Adam Smith's "invisible hand" to solve our problems through pursuit of profit, or is the system deeply and irretrievably corrupt, where academics merely wear their robes in order to qualify for restricted stock options down the line? I didn't like the thought that my Lyme was little more than a profit opportunity for some investment banker who'd befriended a microbiologist with dreams of the riches to come.

Soon thereafter, some professors at Stanford developed a new antibiotic on their own. This was a kind of AI approach to the problem. The headline was: "Screening thousands of drugs, Stanford scientists determined that in mice, azlocillin, an antibiotic approved by the Food and Drug Administration, eliminated the bacteria that causes Lyme disease."

The press release went on to note:

> A new Stanford Medicine study in lab dishes and mice provides evidence that the drug azlocillin completely kills off the disease-causing bacteria *Borrelia burgdorferi* at the onset of the illness. The study suggests it could also be effective for treating patients infected with drug-tolerant bacteria that may cause lingering symptoms.
>
> "This compound is just amazing," said Jayakumar Rajadas, PhD, assistant professor of medicine and director of the Biomaterials and Advanced Drug Delivery Laboratory at the Stanford School of Medicine. "It clears the infection

> without a lot of side effects. We are hoping to repurpose it as an oral treatment for Lyme disease." Rajadas is the senior author of the study, which was published online in *Scientific Reports*. The lead author is research associate Venkata Raveendra Pothineni, PhD.
>
> "We have been screening potential drugs for six years," Pothineni said. "We've screened almost 8,000 chemical compounds. We have tested 50 molecules in the dish. The most effective and safest molecules were tested in animal models. Along the way, I've met many people suffering with this horrible, lingering disease. Our main goal is to find the best compound for treating patients and stop this disease."

"It clears the infection without a lot of side effects ..." That was a pretty strong statement, coming after picking 8,000 strands of chemical spaghetti out of the bowl and throwing them against the bacterial wall to see what would stick. Plus, azlocillin had not yet been tested in humans, so how were the side effects estimated? One way of doing science, I guess. Certainly one path to an exciting press release.

Well, drugs take years to come to market, as we all know, so maybe this will be it one day. However, I did notice that the researchers here again patented the drug and arranged a deal with a biopharma company to "develop" the opportunity. That also at least partially answered my question as to why this research was going on at Stanford, though California is not exactly a hot spot for Lyme infection. Too, when the scientists say, "It clears the infection," they should actually be saying, "It clears the infection in a test tube," since these were in vitro studies. Mind the fine print.

Plenty more researchers, doctors, "functional medicine doctors" (FMDs), and Lyme-curious institutions stepped up to take a swing at the Lyme piñata.

I read about, or "helpful" friends told me about, Rife machines, invented by an eccentric scientist in the 1920s, devices that emitted electromagnetic waves that were alleged to break apart the bacteria (think an opera singer cracking champagne flutes with her highest notes). Oh, and it was also claimed that these machines could break up and destroy malignant tumors. Quite a few otherwise serious people asserted that they "felt better" after Rife treatment. One can't help but remark that the peripheral pseudo-medical world is "rife" with such mysterious approaches.

Some functional medicine doctors took patients to Mexico to inoculate them with malaria, on the theory that the fevers produced by the disease would kill *Borrelia*. On the surface, this strategy didn't seem nutty to me, since it was well known through lab experiments that *Borrelia* (and most other bacteria) are heat-averse (they go static at 101.5°F). One could not help but consider that the fevers produced by the immune system are the body's natural approach to microscopic invasive pathogens, and fevers are typical immune greetings to new cases of Lyme. It made "sense" to me, a layperson. Indeed, I developed a habit of taking extremely hot baths as a technique to at least slow down the replication of *Borrelia*. I raised my body temperature to 101.5°F or more, the level (mild fever) that microbiologists said would have an effect. It did seem to reduce the number and level of symptoms. Nothing to lose here; worst case, my muscles were relaxed and my blood flowed, and I felt better all over from taking baths.

Similarly, induced "hyperthermia" became the basis for a rigorous medical procedure in Bad Aibling, Germany, giving a whole new meaning to the notion of hot baths. Here the patients are sedated while their bodies are slowly heated in a tent. It takes about two hours for the core temperature to reach 107°F. The inventor, Professor Douwes, says the patient's body is left at that temperature for another two hours to kill off the Lyme bacteria. We're talking serious fever here, and the good news claimed is that it will also kill your cancer. At $40,000 per treatment, it had better! Bad Aibling has numerous testimonials—a common feature in this sort of thing—but there are no studies I could find, nor any approvals from the FDA or its European equivalent. One of the largest funders of Lyme research in the US tells a story of her own relief from the treatment, but as far as I know, none of her research grants have been directed to hyperthermia strategies.

Perhaps the opposite would work? If not heat, then what about cold? What about cryothermia? This stone had also been turned over, with the expected hyperbolic statements from its purveyors. The basic pitch is that whole-body cryotherapy "can be used to suppress the Lyme-related inflammation that causes chronic symptoms." If heat won't do it, try freezing the buggers. According to partisans and purveyors of this approach, Lyme is associated with inflammatory cytokines—this we all learned during COVID may be the case in infections; symptoms are a result of "cytokine cascades." According to the freeze folks, extreme cold can not only diminish inflammatory cytokines but also increase *anti-inflammatory* cytokines. I've said a number of times that I'm neither a doctor nor a scientist, but this claim makes me sneeze my milk back into the glass!

So many other untested and unproven approaches to Lyme, including infrared saunas (a cousin to Rife machines)—invisible rays cooking your bugs within (but cooking what else at the same time?)—and hyperbaric chambers were proposed. The theory behind the latter was that intense oxygen exposure would create an oxidative environment hostile to the bacteria; but no proof of this exists, and hardly even any testimonials. Here, too, as is often claimed of these mechanical cures, the great side effect is that it will also kill your cancers. Yay.

OK, I'm a step past skeptical about non-antibiotic approaches to treating the very clever and difficult *Borrelia burgdorferi*. Perhaps I shouldn't be, because the desperation of people feeling that their lives are *over* is serious, and worthy of compassion. But the opportunism of practitioners and companies regarding people who are suffering from illnesses that haven't responded to conventional medical practice is just dismaying. The fact is, chronic or PTLDS sufferers are vulnerable to promises, no matter how unfounded. There is no help to be found!

But lined up by the side of the road are a parade of greasy hucksters ready to accept cash for strategies that are cast to sound scientific, even though none have any basis that would be accepted by even a generous interpretation of what might constitute science: something tested on large groups of diverse humans, tests that can be repeated on additional large groups, results that show clear improvement, no ignored confounders of the results, side effects that are tolerable and acceptable when balanced against the improvement seen.

I'm a bit mechanically inclined, so I looked with hope into these nonmedical approaches, but came away suspicious, skeptical, disappointed, and sad. Simple very hot baths were the most reliable "protocol" I found, and they cost no money. But I'm also persistent and tenacious, and kept looking.

What about herbs? someone said. The Chinese and Indians have used herbs for thousands of years; there must be something in it! Having seen how gullible people are in lining up for modern tools, I wasn't all that ready to think there was "something in it."

Here one guy stood out: Stephen Buhner, not an MD but a "healer" and herbalist, one of these obsessive autodidacts who dig and dig for factual reality, that guy with the long beard whose respect for plants knows no bounds, and who didn't seem to have much of an agenda for his knowledge other than putting it out there and spreading the information. The science background of what he had to say was thin, but *he wasn't selling herbs or herbal retreats.* How refreshing.

I'd never really seen herbs as anything other than an incident of hippie-dom, and the elevation of Native American relation to the world as philosophically better than Western rationalism and material progress. As I read around, though, I found many people of Buhner's type, with a sincere belief that plants—hundreds of millions of years older than humans—had evolved chemical responses to the environment that were tuned and refined. In this zone, I didn't have the feeling that people were in it for the money. So, whether right or wrong, I wasn't being seriously scammed. Too, herbs had been at the center of medicine in China and India for thousands of years.

I was, like anyone, susceptible to anecdotes and analogies and mysticism, but I thought there was something to explore here. Aspirin came from salicylic acid in willow bark, right? A vast number of our medicines came from replications of chemicals found in Amazonian plants, right? Coffee comes from a plant, not a glass carafe. Even Metamucil is just the husks of psyllium seeds. Indeed, as recently as 2015, Professor Tu Youyou received the Nobel Prize for her discovery of the power of artemisinin—which is found in *Artemisia annua* (sweet wormwood)—to cure malaria. And let's not forget the clear efficacy of marijuana!

Stephen Buhner opined that the very best herb to kill *Borrelia* was cat's claw, a woody vine from the Amazon long used to treat various infections, so named for its distinctive large, claw-like thorn that emerged at various points along its viny path.

So I got some cat's claw tincture, with high hopes that it could replace my dependence on telithromycin. I didn't have any clear idea about the right dosage for Lyme—a common problem in herbal treatments—so I just squirted a dropperful of tincture under my tongue, pretty much at any random moment when I could remember to do so. I kind of liked the small sting of alcohol when depositing it in my mouth, but couldn't taste much beyond that. I'm not sure I gave it much of a chance—about a month of undisciplined dosing—but honestly, I felt nothing, nothing at all.

By 2018 the Ketek well was completely dry in the US and in Europe. My guy in the business could no longer bring it back from France. There was no more inventory anywhere, and Sanofi-Aventis announced one day that it had ceased manufacturing telithromycin "for business reasons." I was on my own.

Hot baths didn't seem like enough. I knew that even without new acute symptoms, the Borrelia was in there slowly but inexorably replicating. Like many people with chronic conditions, I remained busy seeking relief and explanations, researching everything about Lyme at credible sources worldwide. (Lyme was global by now.) Leading mainstream researchers had professional seminars posted on YouTube, online social media groups occasionally had visitations from acknowledged experts, and sometimes public television or radio would do a special.

But everywhere it was pretty much the same old story, rote repetition of the known facts without any nuance. I sought salvation with a Google alert on "Lyme treatment," but the landscape of news was barren and impoverished. The lack of progress on the research front was disheartening. After all, it had been only a few years since hepatitis C was literally cured with a 12-week treatment by a new drug developed at Gilead Sciences. The same company had gotten HIV/AIDS thoroughly under control. Great strides had been made worldwide in controlling malaria. Huge efforts were underway to control COVID-19, and at least its spread was fairly well understood. The invisible had been made visible for many microbes. TB was suppressed years ago; polio too. Many cancers had been cured or put into remission by the new class of immune-oncology drugs, like Keytruda. Science can work! Even syphilis had lost the battle to penicillin. Still, there were no breakthroughs for Lyme.

How many times can you read that *Borrelia* is a spirochete bacteria with several stages of life and an uncanny ability to evade the immune system? Or that "it's tick season, so be sure to check yourself and your children after being outside, especially in the woods"? How often would I have to read that a new bite is often but not always accompanied by a bull's-eye rash, and that a course of doxycycline would cure most *new* cases in a matter of weeks? (How much doxy and how long remained a matter of dispute by those in the know.) Or that persistent symptoms might be due to a few persistent organisms or fragments of bacteria that trigger immune reactions, or that for chronic borreliosis, a 28-day intravenous infusion of ceftriaxone would cure "most" people (said the CDC)? Was I in that big scoop of "most," or left outside the responsive swath?

It was all a big downer, but mercifully in 2018–19 I wasn't feeling really obvious neurological symptoms, just inexplicable fatigue that would strike without notice after even the most modest energy depletion. I was busy, too, selling my business to its employees in an employee stock option plan (ESOP). Was I sick, or just weary of all the paperwork and documents I had to master to complete this transaction? (The final closing document ran to 1,500 pages, by the way, a field day for the lawyers.) This, combined with a knee-replacement procedure and recovery, filled the days for a little over a year. That was all over by the end of 2019, leaving me more time to indulge my increasingly consuming hobby of medical research, futile as it seemed.

2020:
COVID Begins

A few stories about a new bug rapidly spreading began to hit the media. We'd never lived through a pandemic, so the idea of a microbe that could soon infect everyone seemed abstract, but the tension was clearly building across society and around the globe. It was both abstract and terrifying. Because of my diverse readings in medical literature, I understood what was happening better than I might have before, yet things you can't see are hard to grasp.

The stories began to emerge in February of 2020 while I was in Jamaica, where my wife and I had gone to rent a little place on the beach and goose our creative juices—not to mention escaping the inimical bitterness of the upstate New York winter. Then, just when we were in transit home in the beginning of March, the US was alerted to the suddenly exploding pandemic of COVID-19. We thought we were just on our way home, but we were *really* on our way home, the home that would become our refuge, along with our Gen Z son, for the next year. On the plane I made a very short poem, fashioned after the public notice signs you see posted everywhere in Jamaica, which I found basic and charming and whose format had stuck with me. Always at the top these 8½ x 11 paper sheets proclaimed "notice" or "important" and then went on to deliver the message. Mine was:

IMPORTANT
Mostly
Invisible

In the evening I called a friend who lived on an avenue in New York City. "It's horrible," she said. "Listen to this. I'm going to put my phone out the window." All I heard were sirens from the street in the night, one ambulance after another.

Finally home, we used the lockdown days as a space for building up skills in the things we loved, whenever it was possible. I couldn't train in aikido; what could be more COVID-risky than a semi-grappling martial art in which you're sweating and breathing heavily on a partner, in a room full of partners also sweating and breathing heavily? I needed exercise, though, and picked up tennis, a sport I'd done in childhood, hoping now to improve enough to get on the court with my wife, who'd suddenly and surprisingly become a tennis addict about 10 years prior.

I doubt my COVID hobby is of much interest to anyone, but it brings us back to the subject of this essay; it segues back. Tennis was great for the pandemic; it was outside, and you didn't have to come within six feet of anyone. Too, I hadn't realized it's a wonderfully technical and formful way of movement (similar to aikido in this aspect, only with a cold and merciless ball between initiation and performance). I could see potential for years and years of learning how to do it just the right way, ideal for the kind of skill acquisition on which I happen to thrive. Plus, it turned out I had a kind of natural ability to make hard serves.

All good; I could find ways to have a healthy, happy life even during quarantine.

ONWARD TO THE HOSPITAL!

Then, one extremely hot day in August, the scene with which I opened this essay: I blacked out on the court, and awakened, bleary, just as the ambulance was pulling into the emergency room parking lot. I was booked, and then catheterized so they could administer the "clot-busting" drug TPA, then sedated and shipped upstairs to intensive care. When I realized where I was, the first thing I wanted to know from the nurse was whether there were any COVID people in the hospital, or nearby. Funny what's top of mind when you return to consciousness. But at that time we all thought we might die from it ... as many already had.

My week in the hospital remains a bit vague in memory, for obvious reasons. Of course, as a purported stroke patient, I went through all the standard tests. Every few hours, it seemed, I would be hoisted onto a gurney to be rolled down a hall with heavy automatic swinging doors and deposited into a chilly room for MRI, CT, CCT, EKG, ultrasound, echocardiogram, transesophageal ultrasound, and finally a stress test with chemically induced heart exercise. Big, high-ceilinged, brightly lit white basement rooms filled with relentless machine hum.

I'll spare you the boring procession of nurses and cardiologists—each of the latter explaining what a stroke is and even drawing little pictures. To each of these cardiovascular specialists I spoke of my long-term Lyme, and Lyme carditis, and the fact that the RBBB they saw on my EKG reads was first identified when I was tested because of severe peripheral neuropathy that was almost certainly from Lyme, since there was no other cause found. From each practitioner I got a blank stare, a look that might as well have said, "not my department."

Then, after I'd spent three or four days in bed, a strange neurologist showed up as I sat with my wife plotting about how the hell I could get out of there. There was no entourage of white-shoes nurses announcing his arrival, no notice an hour ahead of time (everything happens at least an hour later in the hospital), not even much of a knock before he entered the room, where my wife happened to be with me, awaiting the next item on the agenda. He wore a kind of fez-like dark blue hat of a sort I'd never seen before. His face was foreign and unplaceable. Middle Eastern? He wore no scrubs, no official medical uniform, only street clothes and burgundy loafers, which I noticed were rudely scuffed, especially around the pinky toes.

After introducing himself as the in-house neurologist, he launched into a kind of identification speech, explaining in a thick but unplaceable accent that he was a member of an ultra-Orthodox group in Israel, a group whose name I can't remember. "They hate us in Israel," he said. "They discriminate all the time. They kick at us walking down the street." My wife and I nodded and smiled politely, both wondering why he was telling us all this. *This is my doctor? I thought. Is this really my doctor? OK, fine, you're in a radical religious sect in Israel. But what about my stroke?* He didn't even have a hanging name tag.

Given how out of the mainstream he seemed, I tried out my Lyme spiel on him, explaining that I'd first contracted the illness roughly 40 years earlier. Maybe this odd man out would be an interested ear. When I had an MRI for Bell's palsy about 10 years prior, I told him, the scan showed what radiologists called "white matter intensities" in my brain. The radiologist at that time had written that they were characteristic of central nervous system Lyme. I was very interested in this subject, because with all that time in the hospital to think, and a full battery of cardiovascular tests that showed no clots and no evidence of a conventional stroke, I had come to feel that *Borrelia* was still in my brain. But was it growing there, like a kind of dispersed tumor? Was it still colonizing? Had it been gradually taking over during most of my adult life?

Given that he was the first doctor who didn't laugh me off or look the other way, I asked for his card. "I don't have a card," he said. "I just work at the hospital."

Amazingly, he took it upon himself and said he would dig out the MRI from 10 years earlier. This was even more amazing because in our area one couldn't imagine those records would even be stored, and I happened to know that the imaging facility where I'd had the previous MRI was no longer in business.

Surprises never cease—this strange man found out where the images were hiding, and compared them to the present ones. Two days later he showed up again, still wearing that deep blue Middle Eastern fez, to tell me that the *evidence of Lyme in my brain had gotten worse* since the first MRI.

Oh geez, I thought, *what can I do?* He went on: "There was no real evidence of a stroke as we usually see it. No clot. I think what happened is that the infection weakened small vessels deep inside your brain, and the pressure from your heavy exercise made a small vessel or two burst. Then it makes a short circuit, the connections get fried, the information can't go where it wants to go. Everything goes haywire. That's what I think happened."

Many months later I learned from research that cerebral "vasculitis" is a known symptom or effect of Lyme neuroborreliosis (neurological Lyme); it's not in the least bit controversial. I took this news to my cardiologist, who was baffled by the fact that none of the standard tests showed a stroke, although I had, on the surface, many of the signs and symptoms of a stroke. I saw his eyes glaze over, as I'd seen many times from doctors—that lack of interest in anything outside his specialty. I presume Lyme vasculitis must be overlooked in the continuing education seminars most cardio professionals are required to attend.

From the hospital I got a phone number for the Israeli neurologist and followed up, asking him what I should do. He said, as best I could make out through his thick accent, "You need to see a neurologist who also knows about Lyme." OK, I put that on my list.

It wouldn't happen for a while, since after a cerebral event you need to sleep and sleep and sleep as you gradually awaken back into the world you left and the self you had before.

Meanwhile, they let me out of that dreadful hospital room. I had to go back down to the ER to check out and receive discharge instructions. In a small office I sat, staring at the clock whose second hand moved in a disconcertingly jerky motion, while I waited for the doc in charge to come in. He entered with a clipboard. When I caught sight of him, a jolt of emotion and anger lit up my brain.

It was Doctor 1, that same first doctor who fired me in 2002 when I wanted him to consider Lyme as the cause of my burning feet! I wanted to scream at him. "You piece of crap!" I wanted to say. "If you hadn't been such an arrogant ass 20 years ago, I wouldn't be here now!" My restraints were down because of all my brain had been through. I wanted to do him in! I wanted to pound on his chest. I wanted to tell him he'd ruined my life! Previously I said this guy would have a Stendahlian reappearance. This was it. In a sense he had set me up for this exact hospital admission 20 years prior, with his ignorance and refusal to consider anything new. And now he signed off on my release. Not my true, real, and deep release in any deeper sense as a person, just papers from that dump of a hospital.

Home again. I was adrift; in the end with no real stroke, no absolute and certain knowledge that Lyme was still growing in my brain, no treatment of any kind, no screaming revenge on the doctor who could have helped me years ago, could have helped me avoid being right there then. My memory wasn't gone, though. I remembered the advice of that crazy hospital neurologist to go find another neuro who knew about Lyme.

FINDING A TOP GUY TO HELP ME

When I'd rested enough, and recovered enough to contemplate traveling, I found a guy who just might fit the bill, with a practice about two hours' drive from my home. He was cited in many of the research papers on Lyme that were published on the NIH website—you'd see his name and papers over and over again in the research paper footnotes—and he had published many papers of his own. He was both a certified neurologist and an infectious disease specialist. But not just any infectious disease doc. This guy was a leader among the mainstream infectious disease docs who'd studied Lyme. Indeed, he'd been head of the committee that established the official IDSA treatment guidelines for Lyme, the same guidelines that were picked up and parroted by the CDC.

I was excited driving down to the neurological institute of which he was also the director and chairman. I was off to see an *authority*, a Top Guy in the field, a featured speaker at symposia, someone who could tell me for sure whether or not Lyme was continuing to grow in my brain.

We walked down the long hallway to his office together. "I'm reading your book," he said, putting some words into the empty silence between us. I had written several books, so of course I asked him, "Which one?"

"I meant the reports on your case," he said. I had a vision of all the studies, all the imaging, all the blood tests, all the vitals, the MRIs, the CTs, the CCTs, the EKGs, the ultrasounds, the stress test, all the doctors' appointment commentary, together trapped in a heavy black leather pressure cover (no blue three-ring binders for this aristocrat of infection!) with his name embossed on the cover in gold. My book. My "stroke" book. Ready for his dark wood shelf. Would he write up my case for the professional journals?

Once again, the textbook neurologist's examination. It was odd, this guy didn't really look like a doctor, more like a med school professor. He wore a well-tailored suit, a dark tie, clunky brown oxford shoes. His lips were narrow, the sort ready to clearly articulate correct answers. He wore adult glasses with thin metal rims that didn't seem to reflect any light. All serious and very professional, no warm smile, no sense of urgency or hurry, no doubt. I sensed his familiarity with his routine as he ushered me from his executive-desk office into his exam room. The tapping of the little silver hammer, the pricking of the pins, the high A-note of the tuning fork, the bright point of light in my eye, the walking along a straight line on the floor, the hands gently on my neck, turn left, turn right, follow my finger with your eyes, what was the name of your third-grade teacher?

After this ritual we went back to his office, where I noticed the expansive surface of his desk completely empty except for my large "book." I've always been annoyed by clean and well-organized desks, but I felt no rage at this moment—I was almost breathless anticipating his evaluation. I had gotten two disks of my brain MRI to show him, to compare then and now, which he slipped into a computer that was slightly off to the side, and he spent some time peering into the screen at them. From where I sat, I had a side view of the images and marveled once again, as I often had in the past, at the bilateral features of the brain, which came out looking like a colored bird with spread wings as he scrolled through the "slices" of brain that the machine had picked up.

"So," I said, "I came to see you because I want to know if the bugs are still growing in my brain. Do I have to worry about going down again? Will it get worse?"

He opened my "book" to some tabular information, then sat back and made a church steeple with his fingertips. He gave me a deep look directly in my eyes, and his face took on a look of serious authority, with his eyebrows rising; several wavy creases appeared on his forehead.

"I see here they gave you a Western blot test in the hospital," he said, pointing to a series of vertical bars on a graph. His forehead elided from wavy creases to authoritative bilateral lines at downward angles.

"No, you don't still have Lyme," he said. "It doesn't show up on the Western blot blood test they gave you in the hospital. It would be there if you still had Lyme."

I took another tack. "Well, this is a 40-year case; would that make a difference? I couldn't find any studies of such a long case. Would the length of the term here matter?"

"We don't have any data on that. But it doesn't matter. If you don't test positive, you don't have it."

So that was it. No continuing Lyme, nothing further to do, nothing to see here. No suggestions about what to look for in the future.

I left the office unsatisfied, though I thought I should have felt reassured that I wasn't soon going to be shocked by a sudden stroke. I drove home in a kind of numb state. I'd expected more. A diagnosis, a prognosis, a pep talk, a diet, a warning ... something more from this authority, this Top Guy!

At the time, it didn't quite register that he based his opinion on the Western blot test taken from my blood sample. Yet my symptoms, both recent and historic, were mainly neurological. Apparently it did not occur to Top Guy—recall, "neurologist" was one of his credentials—to test for central nervous system involvement.

I adjusted to what had morphed in my mind into a one-off event from which I could just move on. I needed to live again. But the shock of a stroke—it is a literal shock to the brain—doesn't depart on an emotional level just because an expert has ruled out what I thought must be the actual cause. There is a PTSD to it. I could see myself going out to practice serves and falling unconscious next to the basket of yellow balls, no one around to come get me, just a lone man splayed out on the court, unmoving, in the indifferent silence.

Or driving into town, conking out, and ending up wrapped around a tree. Passed out behind the wheel.

How could I go on with this uncertainty looming everywhere?

I thought of hiring someone as a kind of supervisor, someone who could at least call 911. My wife took this as a personal affront. How could I do such a thing? How could I do this to her?

I thought I was pretty rational. I guess it bruised her self-identity as a caretaker of me.

I found myself seeking other causes, first attributing the stroke to dehydration. But the symptoms didn't really match up to what I could find about dehydration, though at the time I had been sweating like mad when playing tennis in the heat for successive days on end. If not dehydration, and not cardiovascular in origin according to my test results (one doc called it a "cryptogenic stroke," a fancy phrase for "we do not know the cause"), and not from Lyme according to one of the world's top experts on the matter, then what was it? How could I leave the house not knowing how it came, or when it might come again, or whether the next time I wouldn't recover? Utter blackness and paralyzed limbs get one's attention.

Little did I know that the "stroke" was a kind of bursting of the dam that had suppressed many symptoms in many systems of my body, what Dr. Aucott of Johns Hopkins has termed *dysautonomia*. Let's just say that's medspeak for "everything crashing." Indeed, one system after another began to break down, commencing with weakening of the small blood vessels of my brain.

2021:
After the Dam Has Burst, a Flood

By the end of the year and into 2021, I started feeling dizzy and unstable all the time, or much of the time. It's a feeling as though I were standing on a floating dock, or standing up on a rowboat on a lake rippled by breezes, sometimes strong breezes, but always breezes. I could stand, but it felt unstable; I could fall if I didn't pay close attention. My house is separated from my studio/home office by a roughly 50-foot, occasionally irregular stone pathway. I'd get up in the morning feeling kind of normal, and then halfway to the studio I'd start to sway inside. I'd have to stop and get my bearings. It would continue, on and on. Soon I'd just lie down in hopes it would go away, but as soon as I got up again, the ground under my feet again became a tilt table on springs.

You might have felt something similar while drunk, or "tipsy." I could carry on a conversation, or walk myself from place to place, or pour myself a cup of coffee, or ponder where and how I could get some relief, but everything felt drained of color and detail. It was like living in an X-ray. The structure was there, but no flesh, no hair, no expansive feeling of excitement or joy, no enthusiasm for the future. Living was more like being a wobbly old milk-wagon horse, knowing where the delivery stops are, but taking no pleasure in it, finding nothing new or interesting in it. Just relief at making it to the next chair or couch. I had to watch where I stepped. Kind of a drunk feeling; even my speech got a bit slurry, as though the nerves connecting to my lips were not quite working.

Next came myalgia: painful, sore muscles and ligaments all over my body, in all the soft tissues, creating a kind of rigidity and loss of flexibility. It was as though my muscles had turned from useful servants into a stiff and uncooperative suit of armor. Aching and sore, like the day after a massive hike up and down a mountain wearing a heavy pack when you haven't even been for a walk in the preceding year.

I couldn't bend over to put on my socks and had to ask my wife for help. It was hard to reach around while on the toilet, too, though we mercifully have a bidet. Putting on a T-shirt became a process of sussing it out on the bed and figuring out how to slip and snake my way into it, rubbing my body on the covers to force the shirt down over the rest of me. Everything was frozen. I'm actually fairly nimble, in part due to a lifetime of aikido practice, but I started making small stumbles, missing a stair tread, bumping into a table leg. My feet weren't going where they used to automatically; each step became an exercise in conscious, intentional movement. Nothing made it worse, and nothing made it better. Every day, upon awakening, there was that ache and rigidity, rolling backward and forward to wrangle myself out of bed.

As you can imagine, this was not a good thing for aikido (our dojo had reopened after the pandemic calmed down), in which I'd been training even longer than I had coexisted with Lyme. Almost half of the practice involves taking on the role of the attacker, who is then thrown down to a semihard mat by a defending partner. Might sound violent, but it's really half the fun, to fall away from danger, or fly through the air and roll out of it like a gymnast. But when every cell of your musculature needs some WD-40, it's not fun any longer. Aikido became a kind of torture or nightmare, because after I was thrown in a technique, I *couldn't get up*! Well, after a while, with some rolling around to find a position where my limbs had a little strength and could work to raise me back to vertical, I could get up slowly, very slowly. Before, I used to just bounce back up to my feet. Also, the movements of aikido are circular. I would try to take class, but would get too dizzy to go on.

Writing and remembering this, it seems to me that, well, there are worse things. It's not cancer; many people are worse off. Right? I guess there are worse things than dysautonomia. Myalgia took away a huge source of joy. It did not seem right that a bite 40 years ago from a tiny insect and an even tinier bacterium inside the tiny bug should take away whatever mastery I had developed over 47 years of training four to seven days a week. I began to see myself as a victim; life dims when you enter victim world. I'd like to say I felt more profoundly and sympathetically the victimization of so many people all over the world who were suffering worse than I, from so many different causes, but I didn't. I was only interested in my own small life, my own damage, and the "off" switch it had flicked on my vitality.

But wait, there's more!

First came the dizziness, then came the myalgia, then came the chills.

This one is a little difficult to describe, but when added to the mix of dizziness and myalgia, it concocted a potent and disabling brew. These were not the same chills you get when you're sick, with alternating high and low temperatures. These were a kind of unhappy tingling primarily across my chest and forearms (those forearms, one of the very first symptoms from 1982). And yet my body said their message was "cold," almost no matter what the outside or room temperature might be—a number I checked regularly, since I no longer felt confident in knowing if the air was cold or not. It would start in the morning and continue through bedtime, so I was uncomfortable with little means of redress each and every day. There was an implied sense of fragility, as if the tingling/chills were just an intro for something soon to come. If you told me this was just a warmup for my body bursting into flames, I would not have been surprised.

What is this feeling of cold but not really cold, this similar-to-cold with no reading on the oral thermometer? It was not the numbness you get in your arm from a pinched nerve or a disordered vertebra. It was not the distended-nipples kind of cold you get when going out in just a T-shirt with the west wind whipping through you. It was a little like the slightly sick feeling you get before liftoff from mushrooms or acid. There was no knee shaking or chattering of teeth. More like the beginning moments of a flu than the flu itself.

Rather than cold itself, or objective, measurable cold, it was more the essence of cold. Isolating, a barrier between self and world. You are not welcome here, says the room, the air, the woods outside, and the sky. If you saw me, you'd not know I was chilled deep inside, with the skin over my core irritatingly electric.

I slept wearing layers: a T-shirt, a wool shirt, and a hoodie, under a down quilt. No matter how warm I made the bedroom. Every night, a cocoon of clothes and covers, hoping to fall asleep. I took lots of hot baths, mostly because by now I was becoming increasingly convinced that the problem was Lyme, no matter what my Top Guy doc said. I remembered that *Borrelia* did not like heat at all, that heat would at a minimum slow down its growth. Made sense to nonscientist me. After all, our immune system produces fevers, high heat, all by itself, as a defense against invasive bacteria.

Hot baths brought some relief while I was in them—I was no longer chilled—but no sooner was I dried off than it was once again time to put on layer after layer and spend my time as a sick person.

This is not a known symptom of any other illness I could find. In isolation it might be called "radiculopathy"—something similar that can be caused by pressure on nerve roots in the spine. This seemed unlikely, with no back issues that I knew of, and the proximity in time to my other symptoms suggested it was connected, as part of a kind of syndrome. But unusual and difficult-to-describe symptoms don't get you very far with medical doctors. (Spoiler alert: I found later there may have been some spine issues after all, but they were still Lyme related.)

Nevertheless, I took my sack of symptoms to the cardiologist, the one whose eyes had said, "not my department," when I'd tried to bring up Lyme to him as a possible lead to understand my "stroke" when conventional testing could show nothing. Even the final write-up said, "no evidence of infarct." No clot, no blockage, no traditional tell-tale of stroke.

"I think you need to see a neurologist," he said. I had been thinking the same thing. He recommended a kind of maverick local guy with impeccable credentials, including UCLA and Johns Hopkins. (He had an unusually strong résumé for our area.)

This guy, I'll call him "Rustic Doc," had a small office in a little town that was a satellite of a large practice some 40 miles away. The receptionist was so warm and familiar I felt like we were old friends. The doctor was big and burly and wore a plaid flannel shirt. There were pictures on the wall of him playing tennis. Maybe I could get somewhere here.

I started talking to him about my history, starting with the big bite in 1982, on to the foot burning, on to the Bell's palsy, the fatigue, the periodic suppression with my savior Ketek. I was talking a mile a minute trying to bring him up to speed on my Lyme life story, all leading up over decades to the cryptogenic "stroke," which by now I was quite convinced was a product of chronic or long-term post-treatment Lyme disease syndrome.

"Whoa!" he said. "Let's try to find out what was behind your event and these sequelae symptoms." That's a medical word for continuing symptoms that are the result of a previous injury or infection. Then he went into the standard neurological intake exam, which by now I had pretty much memorized.

Once again now, from the top. The little hammer on the knee. The tuning fork. The pinpricks here and there. Following his index finger with my eyes as he swept it back and forth across my field of vision. What was the name of my third-grade teacher? What did I eat for dinner yesterday? Who is the president?

At a certain point he looked deep into my eyes with a practiced tone of sincerity. "I believe you feel these things. I really do believe you feel them." I could tell he'd been to a continuing ed seminar where he learned that Lyme patients suffer not only from their Lyme, but from gaslighting and incredulity among medical professionals. Perhaps because you can still get to the doctor's office on your own, perhaps because there is no foam oozing out the side of your mouth, or because you can speak without stumbling, walk without a cane, or read an eye chart, the common experience of Lyme patients is that doctors will first look for everything *but* Lyme to explain the patient's symptoms. They'll want to run tests for multiple sclerosis, for fibromyalgia, for lupus, for broken vertebrae, chronic fatigue, rheumatoid arthritis, thyroid disease, and psychiatric disorders. Actually, Lyme has become known in the research community as the Great Impostor.

He said he wanted me to see an infectious disease (ID) doctor who was a colleague in the larger practice that owned his office. That was fine with me, though even as I was unspooling my tale of Lyme woe to him, I was thinking of Top Guy doc and my failed visit.

The patient presents with a long history of neurological symptoms, Top Guy must have written in his report. Even a layman like myself had learned by then that Lyme can invade the central nervous system, taking up residence in the cerebrospinal fluid, resulting in a diagnosis of Lyme neuroborreliosis. And it could be there without showing up in a blood test. So why in hell did Top Guy doc just send me away? Why didn't he go further and look for neuro Lyme as a cause? I mean, like, neurological symptoms, right?

I'm afraid poor or missed diagnosis of the various forms of Lyme is all too common in mainstream medicine, whether the doctor is widely published in his field or is a GP in a small town working out of an office in a modest, renovated old house. In part, this is because of underdeveloped diagnostics. The best a blood test can do is to tell whether a patient had Lyme at some point in the past. And whether it's an old or a new case, the blood tests are suboptimally accurate, subject to false positives and false negatives. A spinal fluid test might be more reliable for neuro Lyme (while still vague about duration of infection). All a doctor has to do is write a script for a lumbar puncture, a spinal tap.

Anyway, I was relieved and happy to go see another ID guy, even though it meant another round of visits, tests, waiting rooms, all the rest. Annoyance began to build inside me. I was annoyed with myself for putting too much faith in Top Guy doc, who was widely published and respected in the field, because I was not a research project; I was a sick patient. And I was annoyed at this supposed expert for failing to pursue my case to a more certain conclusion, which by now I knew enough to know had a very good chance of being neurological Lyme—especially after I found leading specialists from SUNY Stony Brook in Long Island, a huge Lyme hot spot, leading off their online conference presentations to hospital staff by highlighting "stroke" and "heart attack."

Anyway, I went to this new ID doc, even though I knew he was something of an IDSA drone. Maybe the actual practitioners in the field are more alert than their research leader, I thought.

"It doesn't add up," he said. "No Lyme in your serum [blood] test, but a history of neurological symptoms." Well, this was progress.

"This is an evidence-based practice," he said, rising up. "That's what we do." Not quite sure why he brought that up, but I've become inured to the fact that MDs are not always that normal in personality. "I want you to have a spinal tap, to test the cerebrospinal fluid. It's the gold standard in these cases. If you're positive, we'll do an IV antibiotic for 28 days." *Ugh*, I thought, but he reassured me it would not be painful and there would not be side effects. It seems like humans always forget the side effects. But I didn't forget that Top Guy somehow overlooked the gold standard from his own medical society!

I'd brought a paper on a study done at Yale on Lyme patients with a 20-year history, and suggested that since zero studies had a patient population with infection as long as mine, maybe this would shed at least some light, or help him step off the beaten path. Just trying to be helpful, like with my first doc—the one who fired me.

This one glanced at the pages and tossed them onto the chair next to me. "I'm familiar with the literature," he said, dully, coldly, and checked his watch. He said he'd set me up if I agreed, and that was that. The test was a long needle in my back, but painless, he explained.

Why didn't Top Guy, much higher up the IDSA food chain than this one, set me up with the "gold standard" himself? What can you expect if even a leader in the specialty doesn't do what any practicing professional paying attention would immediately think of?

At this point I was getting kind of desperate for healing, desperate for cure, so I put my head down and kept my mouth shut. OK, OK, stick that needle in my back!

FINALLY, A DEFINITIVE DIAGNOSIS

The system is so slow … so slow. It took at least two months before the spinal tap was arranged. The "tap" involves anesthetizing an area in the lumbar or lower back and spine where there is cerebrospinal fluid (CSF) but few or no nerves. After anesthetizing the insertion point, the doctor inserts a long needle, and the internal fluid pressure is supposed to push fluid up the needle to a receptacle. It happens that in my case the fluid pressure was poor, so they had to insert the needle in various spots, looking for a richer source. All that poking meant that at moments they actually did touch a nerve or two, which made me jump as if from an electric shock. But it wasn't too bad, especially considering the emotional response one naturally has to white coats sticking a needle in your spine.

Slowly, slowly … It took another month before the lab results came back. The neurologist delivered them to me.

"You're loaded with Lyme in your CSF," he said. "I don't think I've ever seen such a definitive test readout. There are eight possible bands on the CSF Western blot, and you have all of them."

Oh geez, I thought, *I have neuroborreliosis. Now it's finally certain, Lyme in my spinal fluid and Lyme in my brain.* I was relieved to finally have "evidence," but still steamed that Top Guy hadn't explored my CSF, only my blood. When you're sick, you want to see the wizard in full, not on a day when he really needs a nap.

There's only one conventionally accepted treatment for a diagnosis of long-term Lyme confirmed this way: 30 days of IV ceftriaxone antibiotic treatment. You can go to one of those rooms where they treat kidney patients, or you can be set up to get the treatment at home, self-administered after training by a visiting nurse. The slow wheels took another month to turn before an oddly loud and unpleasant male nurse showed up to instruct me and bring the first large box of supplies. So, every day I'd shoot up into a PICC line (a catheter that goes to your heart) that had been inserted in the hospital, with a port on my arm to attach the fresh syringes of fluid antibiotic.

Though the feeling of being a "patient" had truly descended, I was optimistic. Here I had an accepted diagnosis, and a known therapy, a major league therapy covered by insurance. Before long I'd be back to normal life, expansive, filled with energy and joy, excited to explore new activities and people, surrendering to the creative process and seeing myself turned inside out, revealed through artwork, rolling around on the aikido mat and swinging hard on the tennis court. I could see the horizon, at last.

The infectious disease doc told me it could take about six months before I'd feel the full effect. That wasn't too long, I thought, after all I'd been through. I'd leave behind that dim state of life, a car with no gas. I'd stand without wavering inside. No more chills. I'd be able to tie my shoes! It would just take some time, that's all ...

* * *

Meanwhile, another symptom that had occasionally been visiting me grew in intensity, grew mighty, and began, like a poison gas, to take over my mind.

Brain fog is right down at the nadir of inflammatory infectious disease symptoms. Basically, you lose your essential self in confusion, with depression and despair arising from that confusion. Brain fog is a mini version of what I imagine Alzheimer's feels like, though with perhaps more self-awareness. You get up in the morning and forget what it was you planned to do. You go into the closet for a pair of socks and come out with underpants. You leave the closet and then go back because you can't remember if you turned out the light. Then you run to the bathroom because you can hear the water spilling over the edge of the tub and onto the floor. You forget what you were going to say. You can't meet deadlines—your mind wandered off in the meantime, and you lost track. You feel weak, and useless, and unable to interact with people because of the energy drain.

Brain fog becomes the kind of capstone or completion factor to an experiential state that can only be described as permanent flu. Every day the flu; every day and all day, it feels like the flu. All flu symptoms except for fever. Every day. From morning till night. ...

It was a complete symptom stack: dizziness, sore and tightly strung myalgic muscles, chills or something like them, fatigue, brain fog interrupting short-term memory, and, inevitably, depression. I could not keep track of things. I could not apply for a renewal of my driver's license. I could not follow directions more than two steps, three if I was lucky. I could get to B, but not to C. A simple doorway chin-up bar sat in its box because I couldn't figure out how to install it—even knowing that my wife had installed one elsewhere, and so had my 20-something son. I bought a fancy office chair and it sat, disassembled, on the floor for months, a pricey pile of chrome and leather, a symbol of my own disassembly.

Like anyone, I'm more comfortable in my life if I have the feeling of progress. Even a nice shower carries with it the feeling of progress. Progress comes from identifying a goal and reaching it, or a task and completing it. There's an energy, a charge, within that brings one to the goal, that drives one to the last step of the task. This is just the normal way of being. From the simplest level of, say, pouring a cup of coffee because your goal is to have a cup of coffee, to the most complex enterprises, like starting a new business. This energy wakes you up, and later advises you to sleep so that you'll have the energy to make progress the next day.

But moving forward in any way was impossible with this symptom set, as was any kind of happiness or positive feeling. I would go to my office or studio in the morning, all set to have a productive day making things and solving problems. But once I sat down to collect myself, my head would begin to feel dizzy, the chills would emerge, my tongue would feel swollen as though sick, and movement of any kind would seem far away from possible. Instead of getting up to begin work, I'd sit back down. The best I could muster was watching a YouTube video or cruising the internet seeking, desperately seeking, some new tidbit of information that would lead to better understanding of this massive stasis or some hope for a cure. I couldn't go anywhere; the prospect of energy expenditure was just too daunting. Would I even remember how to operate the pump to put gas in my car?

Every single day hoping for normalcy, but within minutes of waking, the symptom stack and the sense of illness would return. Many long-term Lyme sufferers have described this state as "debilitating," and there's no better word I can think of. *Paralysis* would work as well. One step and then freeze. The brain fog said, "Aww, fuck it."

It could have been worse. I wasn't vomiting all day long. I wasn't spitting up blood. I could walk, even if I wasn't going anywhere. I could still talk. I didn't have sharp pain that made me crave opioids. I didn't have tremors. I didn't need a wheelchair. My limbs worked; I wasn't physically paralyzed, even though I couldn't get them to do much of anything. It was another kind of paralysis that came from an inability to connect up to the inner energy that drives movement from here to there, but essentially has the same effect or result.

This must be the reason why so little effective research into the causes and cures of Lyme has been done. While the symptoms may be debilitating, they aren't fatal, and they aren't acute or gross (though some patients with severe Lyme arthritis might disagree). All that, plus the fact that the pharmaceutical industry hasn't found a way to profit from what's been called "the silent epidemic." But it is a horrible way to live, a way with no prospects, no sense of possibility or future improvement. You lose personality; you despair of the next symptom or the next attack. You wonder if you're going to die this way. You have no joy. You're clinically, hormonally, chemically depressed. Though they say Lyme isn't fatal, you have the feeling that it is slowly destroying your system, that your light will grow weaker and weaker like an old flashlight in the back of the closet, until you're just a small, dull point of life ... just barely alive.

By this time, because of COVID, we'd all learned the phrase *cytokine cascade* to describe the onset of symptoms, and the accretion of symptoms upon symptoms, in the immune response to microscopic pathogens. I read more about this process, and studied it, and came to see that the symptoms of COVID are, except for the pulmonary locus, very similar to the symptoms of Lyme. (This has become a common standpoint and starting point in medical research by now, a view that the two are related.) Cytokines, just to establish what the jargon means, are internally produced proteins or substances made by many different cells that have an effect on the immune system, generating activities of tissue repair. This is true whether the cells or messages that generate cytokines are cancerous or harmed by bacterial or viral invasion, or even by physical injury. So, when there's damage, cytokines are called forth to activate the immune system. There's even a complex known as "cytokine release syndrome" (a.k.a. hypercytokinemia, a.k.a. cytokine storm syndrome). The syndrome will be familiar to anyone who has a malignant cancer, COVID, Lyme, a bad flu, or even the common cold:

—fever and chills
—nausea, vomiting, diarrhea
—dizziness or lightheadedness
—headaches
—rapid heartbeat
—"air hunger," or shortness of breath
—fatigue
—muscle and joint pain
—rash
—confusion
—depression

Using all five fingers, I deduced that my symptoms were not really that specific to Lyme per se, but to the cytokine cascade that fighting the *Borrelia* had inspired. It would be the same by any other name, but perhaps comes into sharper focus under the more familiar name of *inflammation*.

The alien invasion inflames you and your body's counter-attack. And it's not so much the "bugs" that bring you to your knees, it is *your own immune system*!

The immune system is so focused on destroying invaders that it has trouble regulating itself. An invader, whether a toxin or a bacterium, is something like an itch. From within, releasing a death squad of cytokines, the immune system scratches it. And scratches it. And scratches it some more, to be sure the danger is done. Meanwhile, the skin turns red from abrasion. Whatever's caused the itch has spread. Perhaps blood has been drawn, opening the body to yet more invasions. What was a natural healing response spirals out of control, and the host—you, or I—becomes even sicker.

I mentioned before that as Michal Tal from MIT succinctly put it, "Your immune system is extremely powerful. Your immune system can kill you." The symptoms are not the disease, in terms of your own experience. The immune response is the disease, really. Symptoms may vary depending on the particular microbe that's triggering immune response, but the menu is essentially the same for most infectious illness. The problem with Lyme is that *Borrelia* has uniquely evolved to evade our immunity weapons. Through a process known as "antigenic variation," *Borrelia* is essentially able to cloak itself and become imperceptible to immunity processes that would otherwise destroy it. Because it is so evasive, the immunity machine keeps revving higher and higher, trying and failing to vanquish the intruders, producing more extreme and persistent symptoms. Even a handful of surviving microbes can still trigger the cytokines, whose rational function should be to kill and then stop killing. But once put in motion, the immune response tends to stay in motion. A microbiologist said to me, "Cytokines—we need them, but they can overdo."

So I read and thought about the cytokine cascade while dosing up with my IV antibiotic, while waiting for my own cytokines to calm down as the antibiotic killed the *Borrelia* that had inspired them.

I realized that the elements of my state *felt* like a cytokine cascade in my body. Symptoms would arise without triggers, and arise spontaneously throughout the day, as if there was a hidden process to which I wasn't privy and with which I had nothing to do. On any given day in my case, first would come the dizziness, then the chills, then brain fog, followed by weakness, then muscular tension and dispersed pain, next confusion and a loss of focus, including inability to conceive of the next step, and then fatigue, and finally just quitting and a refusal to go on. The stack might vary in sequence, but it was still the same stack.

A month after the IV infusion was over, it seemed as if things were getting better. My eyes, which had grown dull in feeling, began to feel as though they were opening in the morning. Instead of a sense that there was some kind of dull membrane enclosing my eyes, it felt as though air was flowing around them, and under my eyelids. The colors and shapes of the world around me grew brighter and more well defined, a literal increase in focus.

A small seed of optimism began to sprout. Instead of sleeping in a T-shirt, wool shirt, and hoodie under a down quilt, I was down to just a T-shirt and wool shirt under a winter blanket. To be sure, I needed to get 9 or 10 hours of sleep to feel these improvements, but things were, it seemed, a little better. Could it be that my nightmare of diminishment was over? Might I soon stop shrinking into a smaller and smaller world? Would I soon be able to join the land of the living? I saw that IV ceftriaxone might be my savior.

Life returned. For the first time in ages I wanted to go out to a movie with my wife. We talked about going on a short vacation retreat at a nearby spa, though I still wasn't certain I could go on even an hour's drive and sleep in a strange bed. I slept and slept, and awakened now with the beginnings of that feeling of enthusiasm for the upcoming day that had been my baseline in the past, my steady state.

It was still just an outline, but it was there. How I'd longed for that familiar feeling!

I began a calendar recording my improvements, heading for that tantalizing six-month end point the ID doc had told me would be the end of the nightmare. It was now early spring of 2022, 20 months since I went unconscious on the tennis court, and more than a year since I began to feel the muscle stresses of myalgia and the disorientation of dizziness. Ahh, normalcy was possible! And why not? I'd worn the IV line for a month and shot up the drugs every day, religiously. There was a cure, I was almost surprised to find. A good one, certified and paid for by insurance.

Those green shoots proved tender, though. Like the sproutlings that appear on top of a recently cut tree limb, they were fragile, intolerant of the first sharp change in the weather, and unable to grow beyond their initial size, unable to draw forth enough nutrition to keep going and grow another branch. I sensed change, I sensed progress, though it was still hardly full health. Yet the myalgia had relented enough to permit me to put on my socks and tie my shoes. That was indeed a positive marker. With feelings a mix of certainty and hope, I looked forward to relief from all of it.

Yet over the following months I found that the initial changes were not followed by more. Yes, the myalgia had relented some, the chills were less, even the dizziness was less, and there were days I could go without putting myself down for a nap. But the level of improvement was not much. It was like laying a thin pillow over a scream. The scream was muffled, but still there, still clearly there.

The day for my six-month follow-up with the ID doc arrived. I told him the expected six months had passed, and though I was a bit better, it was only a bit; it was minimal. In sum, I said, I still felt sick every day. I'd regressed from the initial improvements toward my prior state. To grade it, instead of a superbad flu, now it felt like merely a bad flu, without the super. I felt it could even revert and get worse. It was fragile. Hot baths and long sleeps helped me feel better, I told him, but the treatment had not proved effective enough. I might have two or three relatively normal hours in the morning, but soon enough I was once again incapacitated.

"It can take up to a year to feel the effects," he said flatly, with a knowledgeable tone.

"But before you said it would take up to six months," I replied, trying to restrain any accusatory tone in my voice.

"Well," he said, "there are cases where it could take a year to have full effect." Oh, lame.

"You mentioned that you have an 'evidence-based' practice, that's what you do. You treat based on data, right? Do you have any data on the response of a 40-year case?" I knew there were no relevant studies.

He just shrugged, both palms up, as if to say life can be full of mysteries, and took out his laptop to make another follow-up appointment for me.

Fast-forward to the next 6-month follow-up, which was actually a 12-month follow-up from the time I'd finished my IV infusion. In the meantime my neurologist had grown engaged over my lack of progress after the antibiotic shock and awe, which presumably should have worked by then. He said he had become concerned that the infection had been "improperly treated." This took me aback, as it sounded in English as though he was disrespecting the infectious disease doc of his own larger practice, though I subsequently learned this is just medical jargon for "the drug didn't work." Presumably in a continuing quest to investigate any *other* possible causes for my symptoms, he had me undergo MRIs of the upper and lower levels of my spine. (He was, after all, a neuro, not an ID doc.)

The MRIs brought new insight into my case—I can't really explain why they weren't prescribed earlier. MRIs don't necessarily show the specifics of a problem, but they do show where there are areas of concern. Recall the earlier brain MRIs I mentioned that had areas of punctate "intensity" in the brain white matter, which were described as typical or characteristic of neurological Lyme. In the image, there are moments of "light" where there are masses, or blocks ... or inflammation.

According to these scans, there was exceptional inflammation of my brain stem as well as in various locations of my spinal cord meninges. The meninges are membranes that protectively wrap the spinal cord, providing insulation from foreign invasion as well as support to keep the nerve and its branches in place. Of course the spinal cord and its meninges are the key parts of the central nervous system (CNS), controlling almost everything important in the body: movement, vision and the other senses, emotions, communication, life as we know it. Having had several friends come down with multiple sclerosis, I knew a little about the impact of a damaged CNS, and it was not a happy slice of knowledge. *Oh shit*, I thought, *do I have MS? Was it really MS all along?*

I asked the neuro. "No," he said, "MS has a different look. It's not likely in this case." Well, that was a relief. But I wanted to know more, so I called the radiologist who'd read my scans. He called back right away, which was a surprise. I guess radiologists never really see patients, so he was happy to get involved in the human behind the images.

"Is the inflammation you noted normal or extraordinary? Do you see a lot of it?" I asked him.

"I've been in this area for eight years now," he said. Recall that in our area of the Hudson Valley, Lyme is endemic. "This is really the worst I've seen."

I took this conversation back to my neuro (wondering a bit why he hadn't had the same conversation with the radiologist himself).

"You have Lyme meningitis," he said. "It's definitive. It could be the cause of most of your symptoms." I realized that the Lyme bacteria had colonized my entire nervous system, not just my brain and cerebrospinal fluid. Well, that made sense; if it was in the fluid, why not all the tissues that touched the fluid too?

I left his office with my head drooping low and stopped off at a deli on the way home to get a doughnut. I felt like there were not enough doughnuts in the deli case to soothe my sense of doom. I wanted to open my throat and stuff it full of jelly doughnuts until it could hold no more. I was crazed, and moved on from the jelly to the cider to the glazed. Give me sugar! Give me dough! Wash it down with Coca-Cola!

END OF 2022:
Treatment Failure

A raised level of panic set in. The mild improvement I'd gotten from the IV infusion was far from a cure, and my diagnosis had now become more acute, more official, more threatening. I was indeed doomed, it seemed. The symptoms were back, if not in full force, then at 90%. I was still sick—as far as I could see, nearly as sick as before. Feeling something like a cornered animal, I cast about in my mind for some way out of the maze, but could see none. Still my brain responded with a refusal to give in.

I had to admit that the IV antibiotics had had some effect, even if it was minor and disappointing, and the initial progress had faded. But I've typically been the kind of person who believes that if a little does a little good, then a lot will do a lot. So hey, how about another round of shock and awe?

Maybe the first course was just not enough. Let's hit them again! I resisted the information I found in research that very long courses of antibiotics actually don't show additional improvement, at least in cases involving spirochetes, like Lyme or syphilis. Depth or intensity is more important than duration. Indeed, one unrefuted study on this issue was done by none other than Willy Burgdorfer, the very scientist who discovered Borrelia as the source of Lyme, and for whom *Borrelia burgdorferi* is formally named. I kept this info to myself. I'd settled in my mind to pitch the ID doctor to prescribe another round of IV, kill the buggers while they were weakened—so I wasn't going to let on what I knew.

The one-year point from the original IV had come around. I'd complained that nothing much was happening after the six-month period following that IV, though it was supposed to take effect within six months, and then another six months, and ... nada. The year had passed, and, essentially, the treatment just had not worked. I pressed him to try another round of IV. He was reluctant, throwing back to me the fairly conventional and accepted knowledge that another round wouldn't do any good and could prove harmful. (Darn, he knew the facts.) He again waved his flag that his was an "evidence-based practice" and there was no evidence from studies that going back to the antibiotic large-scale munitions would help. He looked at his watch. I felt sick inside at the prospect of no more help. I felt weak. Knowing what I knew from research, I was unable to argue, unable to suggest any alternate path.

"Can't you think of something?" I asked, or maybe I should say begged. He looked at his watch again.

"There's nothing more we can do for you," he said flatly. I heard it echo in my mind, like sound reverberating in a tunnel. "There's nothing more we can do for you."

I sat there, stunned, as he gathered up his papers and rose to leave. He said nothing further. No "good luck," no "let's set a follow-up appointment," no suggestion to see a different specialist. "I'm sorry," he said again, turning back to me as he entered the doorway, "there's nothing more we can do for you."

I translated this into common speech: "*Too bad you're screwed for the rest of your life. I have other patients to see now.*" I realized I might die like a shrunken beast, with brain fog, joyless, depressed, unable to progress and move forward, dizzy, with chills and aching muscles, no hope of inner growth or learning, no fun, no making high-energy intimate connections with my wife or any other people, just sleep as my only source of respite.

Gong. Gong. Gong.

I went home, digesting what was not exactly a death sentence but something fairly close. A death-in-life sentence. I saw myself as an old man in loose trousers and a rumpled white T-shirt, sitting in a rocker on a porch in a quiet town, seeing my lively life as it could have been, instead just dull and perseverating over and over: *nothing turned out as I thought it would.*

Damned ticks! Damned microbes! Damned nature! All of it!

2023:
The Twist

The life lessons of my life have mostly centered on resilience and tenacity. One foot goes in front of the other. Training in aikido means falling down and getting up again thousands and thousands of times. Managing investment portfolios depends on recovering from losses you didn't cause and over which you had no control, coming back again and again, day after day. My spirit is in good measure defined by a craving for the sense of progress and the acquisition of new skills; getting there means feeding and pumping up tenacity. There are some sweaty old saws that apply, such as one from an old yoga guru I used to like: "We must learn to live in two worlds: the world of inspiration and the world of perspiration."

Anyway, let's just say that the verdict from ID doc was devastating, but I couldn't stop trying, no matter how silly and futile the effort might be. I just couldn't stop, even if it was crazy or far out in left field. The allopathic door now seemed closed. I could try the woo-woo route. Why not? I refused to contemplate life as I was living it for however many years remained in my diminishing life. I did not want to die debilitated.

Reviewing all the research I'd done, I thought back to a study done by Johns Hopkins and first reported in 2020 in *Frontiers in Medicine*, with Jie Feng and Ying Zhang as lead authors: "Evaluation of Natural and Botanical Medicines for Activity against Growing and Non-growing Forms of B. *Burgdorferi*." (https://www.ncbi.nlm.nih.gov/pmc/articles/PMC7050641/)

I dug it out and read it again and again, in hopes there might have been some great promise that I missed the first time around. Honestly, I thought I might be merely going through the motions, because at some point, perhaps just after that period when Ketek disappeared from the scene, I had tried cat's claw, one of the botanicals that the functional medicine folks seem to generally agree is good for Lyme, and I'd gotten nothing. It had seemed strange to insert this alcoholic tincture under my tongue, but I'd performed the ritual, hoping for an effect. We're used to taking the right drug and feeling at least some effect after a few days, but the herb didn't do anything for me. I took down most of an entire bottle (one of those little dark glass bottles three or four inches high), then put the notion of cat's claw on a dusty shelf. After this dud, it didn't seem to me that there was much promise in botanicals.

Nevertheless, when you're told "there's nothing more we can do for you," your horizons open up a bit. I took another look at the substances in the Johns Hopkins study; if they were going to be an option, I didn't want to wind up with liver or kidney failure because of some dumbass and panic-driven experiment. The first thing I wanted to know was whether there could be bad side effects if I tried them—my business life was as a risk manager, after all. I've found that one of my biggest problems, and in our society in general, is forgetting about the side effects. The brain seems to be designed to get excited or optimistic about the imagined upside or potential solution to a problem, but that very excitement often dampens any thoughts of what could go wrong. Dreams are a lot sexier than risks.

Anyway, using my investment manager brain to look for risks, I delved into what was known, positive and negative, about these botanicals. I had time, since there was "nothing else they could do." On a side note, let's dispense with the jargon and professional euphemism. *Botanicals* sounds quite academic, and I like to use the term to gain credibility. But really, what we're talking about here is HERBS! That's right. Herbs.

Don't snicker—there's a long history here, in many cultures other than ours, and even some slightly lost uses in our own society. This zone is not just for beaded and headbanded acolytes of religions conducted in other languages. We're already kind of herbal. We're a coffee and tea culture; those are some of the most powerful and effective herbs on earth. Right? Coffee doesn't just come from a glass pot. It's a bean. Tea is a leaf or a root. We're not averse to botanicals, just not attentive. I found myself going up the learning curve, learning about so many plants and their medical uses in other cultures over centuries and centuries. It was fascinating. I started becoming a bit of an Herb Guy.

Rereading the study, I caught nuance in the text that I'd missed the first time around. In the introductory paragraph the authors make reference to "anecdotal reports on the use of herbal extracts." "However," they go on, "it is unclear whether the effect of the herb products is due to their direct antimicrobial activity or their effect on the host immune system."

That's so circumspect I just have to restate it in English: "We wanted to know whether any of the herbs [botanicals] are actually bactericidal to *Borrelia*. Do they kill the bug? Or do they trigger or help the immune system in its own natural efforts at microbicide?" Implicit in this is a common or accepted notion, a presumption, that herbs are supportive to the immune system or work in tandem with it. This is a pretty safe restatement because, as the authors point out, herbs have been in documented use for thousands of years. And there's been at least some attempt at scientific study of most of them, the results of which I'll summarize here:

Plants contain chemically active substances that are anti-inflammatory.

That's really the starting point. Someone in the back of the room raised a hand to counter, "What about poisonous plants?" Well, OK, just don't eat those. Otherwise, plants contain phytochemicals, such as polyphenols, alkaloids, flavonoids, and terpenes—all features that cool down inflammation—and pretty much all plants contain these to one degree or another. Are they as good as anti-inflammatory drugs from the Big Pharma companies? Maybe not as strong or as quick, but usually without harmful side effects. They are still NSAIDs. They are nature's aspirin—which itself originated as a concentration and purification of the salicylic acid found in myrtle and willow.

And what is inflammation? It is what happens when the immune system goes into action, a kind of biological version of unintended consequences. The NIH tells us, "Inflammation is part of the body's defense mechanism. It is the process by which the immune system recognizes and removes harmful and foreign stimuli and begins the healing process." We experience inflammation as symptoms. Infection doesn't cause symptoms; it causes the immune system to take protective action, and that action is what results in the symptoms we feel. So symptoms are a kind of second-order effect.

Based on the premise that herbs are anti-inflammatory, and accepting that as fact, the study proposed to look at the activity of the herbs separately and outside the human body, with no immune system present to confuse the issue of efficacy. I was fine with what I thought of as the bonus addition of anti-inflammation. But never mind all that invisible stuff. I wanted a cure, not a lesson in immunology. How could I get cured without causing another illness at the same time?

The authors introduce their study—the first and only lab study of its type, as far as I can determine—as a way of looking deeper into "anecdotal" reports on the use of botanicals for treating patients with post-treatment Lyme disease syndrome with persisting symptoms. A meta-analysis they cite (this is a review of all prior work by others) suggests that 63% of patients experience at least some persistent symptoms after treatment. I just hate the claimed precision and exactitude. And it also seems like a high number. Maybe it's more like 50%, maybe it's 75%, who cares? Many studies, they assert, have shown that "*Borrelia* is capable of persisting in diverse tissues across a variety of animal models despite aggressive and prolonged antibiotic therapy."

They then step away from the standard track to look at other approaches that have been suggested and used outside the mainstream medical protocols. But, they go on to repeat, "*it is unclear whether the use of herb products is due to their direct antimicrobial activity or their effect on the host immune system.*" I italicize that statement because it is important, especially if you believe that disease *symptoms* are the result of immune system processes—which I believe isn't a controversial position. If there is an invader, the various immune responses are triggered, inflamed. If the invader is destroyed, the immune system can retreat back into its calm burrow, its waiting state.

In any event, in a laboratory setting (in vitro), they tested 12 commonly used botanicals (of the sort suggested by Stephen Buhner, for example). Of the 12, the top 6 in the list below showed at least some antimicrobial activity, meaning they either killed or reduced test tube populations of *Borrelia*. I gave them a **Y**.

—*Cryptolepis sanguinolenta* (Ghanaian quinine) **Y**
—*Juglans nigra* (black walnut) **Y**
—*Polygonum cuspidatum* (Japanese knotweed) **Y**
—*Artemisia annua* (sweet wormwood) **Y**
—*Uncaria tomentosa* (cat's claw) **Y**
—*Scutellaria baicalensis* (Chinese skullcap) **Y**
—Stevia
—Andrographis
—Grapefruit seed extract
—Colloidal silver
—Monolaurin
—Peptide LL-37

The bottom six (stevia, andrographis, grapefruit seed extract, colloidal silver, monolaurin, and peptide LL-37) were duds. These, often claimed by alternative doctors to have a beneficial effect, proved to have *zero* noticeable activity against *Borrelia*. Now, just because something has an antimicrobial effect in vitro doesn't mean it will have the same effect in vivo, in the human body. But to be sure, it makes no sense to think that if something *can't* impact *Borrelia* in a test tube, it would by some mysterious means have such an effect within the body.

Too, they performed the same tests with the standard antibiotic treatments as a comparison, which puts the successes into perspective. If the botanicals were not as good as or better than antibiotics against Lyme in an experiment, why bother to go forward? If they were better, then there's reason to dig deeper. But no worries; the effective botanicals were better than the standard antibiotics at killing *Borrelia*.

In the image on page 118 from the results of their in vitro tests, we can see how much *Borrelia* bacteria survived treatment in a bath of tinctures made from the top six botanical performers. Each light dot represents stained Borrelia when seen in fluorescence microscopy. Different intensities of tincture are represented by the percentages at the top of the image. If there are a lot of light dots, that means many bacteria survived. The fewer the dots, the more effective and bactericidal the solution. In this case the bacteria were grown for 7 days, then treated for 7 days, then "washed" of the extracts and resuspended in growth solution for 21 days—so what's shown is both the effectiveness of the products in killing *Borrelia* and the durability of the treatment. We'd see more light dots if the bacteria grew back within 21 days.

So, more dots is a worse outcome. Fewer dots is better.

Of note here is the poor performance of doxycycline, the mainstream drug of choice for a new case in which the bacteria are in the bloodstream and in a growth phase. See how bright the doxycycline box is? That means by 21 days after treatment the *Borrelia* were still alive, presumably still replicating. Perhaps they were weakened, perhaps enough for the innate immune system to destroy them, but even if that's the case, the doxycycline was not nearly as potent as several of the botanicals, especially *Cryptolepis*, a scrambling shrub from Ghana known to be effective against malaria.

One by one I researched the herbs found in this study to check about toxicity. To save some time, I focused on four with the best anti-*Borrelia* performance in their tests. I was thinking if these were safe, they would be candidates for what I had come to the edge of deciding would be my personal adventure as a human guinea pig. The study used petri dishes or test tubes for in vitro testing. I would become the in vivo extension of their work.

1% Cryptolepis 60% EE

1% Black Walnut 60% EE

1% Cat's Claw WE

1% Japanese Knotweed 60% EE

1% Sweet wormwood 60% EE

0.5% Cryptolepis 60% EE

0.5% Black Walnut 60% EE

0.5% Cat's Claw WE

0.5% Japanese Knotweed 60% EE

0.5% Sweet wormwood 60% EE

Scutellaria barbata 1%

Scutellaria baicalensis 1%

Juglans nigra fruc 1%

Doxycycline 5 μg/mL

Drug free control

Cryptolepis—Also known as Ghanaian quinine, a scrambling shrub whose root concentrate has been extensively studied and widely used in Africa as a treatment for malaria. Might want to be careful with the active ingredient—cryptolepine—in pure form, but even a multi-gram dose is unlikely to cause problems.

Black walnut—Various polyphenols and vitamins, polyunsaturated fatty acids, cardio- and vascular-protective. Quite tannic, but no known research findings on toxicity. Perhaps best at limited duration of usage. (Though I sure like walnuts!)

Japanese knotweed—An invasive species despised by ornamental horticulturists and gardeners, but one of the best sources of resveratrol, which is well researched as an anti-inflammatory and protector against various chronic diseases and is positive for the gastrointestinal tract, with no negative side effects reported at 1.5 to 2 grams per day (4 cups of tea from powder equivalent).

Sweet wormwood (Artemisia)—Tu Youyou won a Nobel Prize for discovering the efficacy of *Artemisia* as a treatment for malaria (a spirochete protozoan parasite). More potent than many other herbs (base for the creation of absinthe, among other things). My takeaway was, go easy on dosage.

Since there's so little clinical research of the sort you might see for an FDA-approved drug on these (except for *Artemisia*), any use of them for my purposes was going to be pretty experimental. They have been studied enough to suggest that anything other than a massive dose was not likely to cause harm. Of course a massive dose of anything—even doughnuts—is likely to cause at least some harm to the body. Also, because this is a dark, alternative area in the eyes of modern science, it was very difficult to determine the correct dose, beyond the standard dosing described by the herbal purveyors themselves.

How much to take? Ramp it up? How much would be too much? Or too little? And where to get the botanicals that are what they're supposed to be, with a good count and good price? These questions of proper dosage and sourcing were difficult to answer, and perhaps are not fully answered. The Johns Hopkins study, however, did provide the name of the researchers' supplier, so that was a start.

Still, I had decided to go into this knowing there were open questions. Importantly, my alleged "decision" was not really a decision in any normal sense of the word. Since there was nothing more that conventional or allopathic medicine could do for me, and since I was pretty sure the herbs would not kill me, I really had nothing to lose. There were some studies that suggested that a dose for someone my weight could be 10 grams or more—that's a lot, a large margin of error, I thought.

I was miserable, and made even more so by the knowledge that the conventional treatments had failed. It was like having a bad flu every day, I reminded myself, every day for three years. The chills and the aches, losing control of my cognition, lacking in energy to interact with anyone, unable to travel even 10 or 20 miles, crawling back into bed just hoping all the last years of my life would not be spent this way. Not to mention the headline symptoms over the years—peripheral neuropathy, facial palsy, photophobia, cryptogenic stroke.

In a position of weakness, you accept some risks, risks that might not even be all that serious. I could be wasting my time if they didn't work, but I'd already wasted so much time. ...

INTO HERB WORLD

I have mixed feelings about expert authority—you've already seen that—nevertheless I decided to go see a functional medicine doctor who'd have some experience with herbs and could provide some guidance regarding dosage and sourcing. It happened that the president of the national functional medicine group focused on Lyme had an office in my area, and I'd heard his name quite often over the years, never in a bad way. Actually he was another Top Guy, just in the alternative sphere. So I set up to see him, feeling pretty good that I'd have professional mentoring in my new herbs journey. I hadn't started taking any yet, so this was just an information safari.

It started out a bit spooky. While his office was a 45-minute drive from where I live now, it turned out to be located on the same road as my farm from the 1980s where I was bitten that sultry summer, all alone with chills and fevers. In fact, as I walked into his building, I stopped and could literally see the edge of my old property, triggering a fast-forward reel of memories. Strange, it's as though my possible cure was doing business right next door all along!

I knew that building, an old brick former factory amalgam of multiple small offices. Climbing up the stairs (no elevator here!), I faced a long hallway of small alternatives, a counterculture cornucopia. Following along a somewhat threadbare carpet, there were door signs for a psychotherapist, a chiropractor, a local newsweekly, a Rife machine service, a small Pilates gym, yoga lessons, a county farmers' co-op, an astrologer, a peace retreat travel agent, another psychologist, a family lawyer, a circus arts teacher, a budding tofu ice cream alternative company, an acupuncturist, and a guitar teacher. Many of the doors had handwritten 8½ x 11 signs scotch-taped above the doorknob with notices about vacation closures, or new hours, or the location to which the business had moved. Each door had a number, preceded by "suite."

My new Top Guy's office was a little better than I expected. It looked kind of normal; leather chairs with wooden arms, a reception desk behind sliding glass doors. Plain fake wooden paneling on the walls, a burbling jug with plastic faucet for water (little paper cups in a stack).

Signing in, first I had to pay the cash, just like with Woo-Doc, 20 years prior. Call this one Woo-Doc 2. There was a big upfront for the initial consultation, then slightly smaller sums for follow-up; I was asked to commit to at least three follow-ups if I wanted to see the doctor.

Soon enough I heard my name and went into a fairly standard examination office to sit and wait. By and by, Woo-Doc 2 came in, wearing a long white coat, a white coat that fell way below his knees and seemed formal, almost ceremonial—an official (was it too long?) coat of authority. He gave me a cursory physical exam, including a good long look at my tongue and the feeling of many pulses in various places. I'd brought my most recent blood tests, which he perused as expected. Then he stood up to give me a little talk about what to expect. When he rose, I noticed that there was a narrow dark brown stain running six to eight inches down his white coat. Something had spilled. He was mid-60s, with thinning hair, rimless glasses on his nose, and a hidden belly pushing out the coat at his waistline. But that stain! It seemed like the mark of a loser. I'd come for a Top Guy, yet he was stained and mortal, with no spare white coat.

Oh, the magic was kind of gone. Still, I'd driven a ways to come get his expert knowledge. And he did seem to nod knowingly when I described my various symptoms. A little wry smile crept across his face when I pointed easterly toward my old farm and told him I was first bitten "right next door."

Then I told him I'd come to see him because antibiotics had failed, and I'd become interested in a botanical approach after reading the Johns Hopkins study, which had come out about three years before. In his eyes there was no evidence of recognition. "You know," I said, "the study they did on herbs and *Borrelia*?"

He nodded in the way that people do when they don't know what you're talking about but believe they can figure it out from context if you keep talking. "I know it was in vitro," I said, "but I don't think I have any other choice. So I came for your expertise in the products."

He kept nodding but added no further comments, and I realized then that he was not aware of the study at all. *Oh geez,* I thought, *this guy's the president of the association of doctors who use the alternative approach to Lyme, and he hasn't seen the single most important piece of scientific research in his specialty since Lyme was first discovered!*

I saw a sign in my head that read "dead end." As much of a letdown in its own way as my meeting with the allopathic Top Guy a couple of years earlier, if perhaps with a tad less arrogance from the expert.

When the consultation was over, Woo-Doc 2 led me by the hand, literally led me by the hand, to the nicest room in his suite—where he sold the herbs from a glass display case. He gave the attendant a "script" for the tinctures he thought I should take, but had no usage instructions for me.

But there were two moments of interest. First, he confirmed what I'd gleaned from research, that the herbs are best taken in tincture form; they're more concentrated that way, and when you take the drops under your tongue, at least some goes more or less directly into your bloodstream rather than having to fight its way out of your gastrointestinal tract.

Second, he asked me to get a second set of bloods. One script to go to the normal labs that all the doctors use, and one to a secret lab in California where I had to take a kit and ship it, but I could only ship it from an out-of-state location, because they weren't approved in New York. Listen, I'm not exactly wholeheartedly in favor of the establishment, medical or otherwise, but I'm not going to drive to Connecticut to send my spit to a mystery lab. Puh-leeze!

Still, there was something interesting, which later was to prove even more so, in the mainstream bloodwork script. He had me take, in addition to the usual, a test for "complement C4a."

I thought I knew my way around the various blood markers of health (I'm that guy who looks up RDW and MCP and bilirubin, all those strange items that doctors love to scan in your charts). I'm not sure I fully understand complements even now, but I did learn that the complement system is our always-on first line of defense against biological attack from bacteria and viruses.

It took three weeks for the results to come back for the complement test, prompting me to wonder if the mainstream labs are even able to do this one correctly. Eventually I got results for all the normal items plus complement C4a, a reading I'd never seen before. Every one of the typical tests showed up as normal and within range, which is basically what I'd seen all my life. (Generally those who know often assert that Lyme doesn't show up in normal blood tests—except those looking for Lyme antibodies, like the ELISA and the Western blot.) I was surprised to see that my C4a was at 4,500, versus the high end of normal at 500. Nine times the high end of the range! Maybe this alternative doc was onto something.

I can't really speak about the complement system intelligently, except to focus on the comments from a search that suggested that if your C4a is high, it means "your immune system is running on overdrive." Well, I kind of already knew mine was; I had felt the continuing symptoms of the cytokine cascade, the cytokine storm syndrome, for years. Still, it was oddly reassuring to know that this could read out quantitatively, that you could put a number on it. What I had been experiencing was real, not some phantasm in my mind. It was good to know, since there's a school of thought among some Lyme researchers, even after the findings of John Aucott, that there's no such thing as chronic Lyme. And many MDs are still skeptical of it, even to this day. OK then, let them argue with the numbers, the numbers in black and white!

Indeed, I went back to my everyday PCP, whom I think of as pretty smart and open-minded, and raised the issue of my C4a being off the charts. She just kind of looked at me with dull eyes and went back to scrolling my results on her laptop. This is what you get, or don't get, from doctors, even in a Lyme-endemic area. Presumably this marker isn't taught in med schools, or in continuing ed conferences. Perhaps insurance companies haven't gotten around to seeing it as a diagnostic tool.

In any event, this high inflammation marker pushed me forward to follow through with my decision to become a test subject for in vivo application of the Johns Hopkins in vitro study. I was reasonably convinced that the herbal tinctures weren't going to harm me. So, even though questions of dosage and source remained open, I went ahead and started squirting *Cryptolepis* (the number one performer) under my tongue. Never mind the strange sound of the name. Ever since the ID doc had told me "there's nothing more we can do for you," I was out in the wild.

A noisy emotional part of me didn't really believe the study; perhaps because nothing (including a brief foray into cat's claw) had worked so far, or perhaps because what I knew of herbs came from counterculture types who claimed that herbs could heal—that I should believe because they said so.

But I wanted to give it a chance, so I marched through the motions and started dosing every morning, using only the amount suggested on the label by the herb vendor. Was this enough for Lyme? Hard to tell, because in vivo research that would mandate a given amount was absent.

It was not a hard process and took very little time. Just squirt some in from the little dropper. I came to like the stinging sensation under my tongue and in my mouth from the alcohol base of the tincture. I came to like the yellow color of the liquid. (*Cryptolepis* roots are also used to make a yellow dye in Africa.) It was, to primitive zones in my brain, as though the yellow contained a magic power, a deep earth wisdom. As I became accustomed to taking it in, I'd dose up three times a day. It wasn't long before I doubled the dosage from the suggested amount on the bottle. Gimme results!

But nothing happened. Like all of us, I'm used to taking aspirin for a headache and having less of a headache an hour later. That's my idea of a drug; you take it and you feel better soon. Shock and awe. Here, weeks went by and I could still feel no effect. Growing depressed about it, I began to sleep 9, 10, 11 hours or more each night, even 12. In sleep, at least, I was no longer reminded of the shrunken being I'd become compared to the self I'd come to know all my life. I slept and slept, hoping the herbs would work, but insisting to myself that I hold that hope close. One day I'd think, *This is silly*. The next day I'd say to myself, *But the study showed this to be better than ceftriaxone and doxycycline*. Then the next I'd remind myself, *Ceft and doxy don't necessarily work on chronic Lyme anyway*. It was the last shot I could think of to take, so I was busy talking to myself.

Then one day, literally on one day, I awakened to an unfamiliar feeling of normalcy. My mind was clear (!). I could remember what I'd done the day before. I knew what I'd previously planned for today. Maybe all wasn't as clear and sharp as I could recall from my prior self, but there was change. This was perhaps six weeks from the time I began taking *Cryptolepis*. *Six weeks*, I thought, *and it's starting to work*. Good God, I never really expected that this shamanistic ritual pantomime calling forth Mother Nature would actually work.

To be sure, it was again just green shoots. I still had myalgia and tight body, I still had chills and dizziness, and plenty of fatigue starting in midafternoon. But my mind, my consciousness, was coming back. The light was coming back on. Perhaps tentatively, perhaps not full wattage, but clearly there'd been a change. Was it placebo effect? I considered that, and indeed I've often done things in my life where I was hoping for at least some placebo effect, even if what I'd done was irrational in the end. Still, it didn't feel like a mirage. I felt *different*!

OMG, herbs! They might work! I reinvigorated my study of all the herbs, going down an herbal rabbit hole. This might not be the place to report all that I learned, but there's a whole botanical world out there. Herbs for digestion, herbs for calm, herbs for weight loss, herbs to thin the blood, herbs to thicken it, herbs for the heart, herbs for the kidneys, herbs for dreaming, herbs for sex.

Do they work? I have no idea, because there is mostly just anecdotal evidence or the fact that they've been used in other cultures for centuries.

Indeed, there is a subunit of the National Institutes of Health (NIH) called the National Center for Complementary and Integrative Health that is dedicated to exploring what's in its name, bringing news of scientific studies about alternative remedies to the general population. You can search any botanicals there. But if you search *Cryptolepis*, you'll be told, "no results found." Nothing to see here. No studies. If, on the other hand, you search ginkgo, for example, you'll receive a platter of conditions that various people have proposed as being helped by the plant, including that it boosts memory; but most studies are reviewed as lacking in definitive results: research seems to suggest that "ginkgo doesn't help with memory enhancement in healthy people, high blood pressure, tinnitus, multiple sclerosis, seasonal affective disorder, or the risk of having a heart attack or stroke."

In the end, for ginkgo and for nearly every other botanical in their database, you'll arrive at this conclusion: "*Some studies of ginkgo in people have been completed, but there isn't enough high-quality evidence to clearly support its use for any health condition.*"

There really is hardly any solid evidence of the sort a scientist would accept about herbs and herbal products overall. Our tax dollars have been put to work, and the answer is always "More study is needed."

So my response to *Cryptolepis* wasn't backed up by any depth of known facts or measurement statistics, except the Johns Hopkins in vitro study. Maybe I was hallucinating this improvement I'd been feeling. Maybe it was really nothing.

Never mind. *I* am the evidence! *I* am the experiment! I'm the one feeling what I feel. I'm the one whose brain is less fogged than it was, whose synapses are connected, whose sense of the future is returning.

OK, the mind can play tricks. I know that. But this first taste of healing inspired me. For the first time, I had a sense that progress was possible, that I could go forward and escape the muck into which I'd fallen.

Since I'm that guy who thinks that "if a little does a little good, then a lot will do a lot," I ordered more *Cryptolepis*, and also the runners-up in the Johns Hopkins study: tinctures of Japanese knotweed, *Artemisia*, and black walnut. Even as I pressed "buy" (you can get these from herb sellers on Amazon), I knew that I risked confounding my experience of *Cryptolepis*, potentially ending up not knowing which botanical was effective if one or more pushed the initial effects forward. But I didn't care. I was sick! I needed help! Whatever, bring on more rescue!

Then I learned patience. In my experience, and so I've heard from other "users," herbs are not like the drugs that have rapid fireworks as they begin to do their job. You have to stay with them. Their effect is cumulative, bit by bit in the body until they reach a threshold point against your infection.

Each day I self-monitored, comparing to the previous day, stamping my state as improved, not improved, improved only a little; improved a lot was pretty much never the case. Only incremental small gains, if any, but these accrued finally to clear lineaments of feeling that had been missing in the 40-plus months before. Forty months; that doesn't sound like a tragedy, but it leans that way when I realized it was on top of the discrete acute events of four decades past, and that it had been going on intensively every single day, every day for all those months, turning my body and brain into a kind of jail cell or cage, a relentless punishment though there'd been no crime.

The improvement was almost like watching a child grow. You see small changes that you hardly even saw in process, until one day a kind of new level or new step in the stairs becomes solidified and defined. Though each day was hardly felt, the cumulation gave me incentive to keep on squirting those herbs each morning, each lunchtime, each evening before bed. I became dependent, ordering more product so that I'd have at least two weeks' inventory and never run out. Like any addict, I was afraid I'd go backward if I ran out and missed even a single day. If the herbs had taken human form and ordered me to bow down in fealty, I'd have been right there on my knees. Typically agnostic in all things, I became herb-religious.

I wished it were like doxycycline, which within weeks can clear a *new* Lyme infection that's still floating in your blood and hasn't yet found succor and a comfy home in your joints or muscles or cerebrospinal fluid or vital organs. I wanted to recover my former self, my active and athletic life, my busy brain encompassing the chaos and order of this unimaginably complex and energetic world. I wanted to laugh at a joke. I wanted to make a joke. I wanted to care about others and get out of the haze and fog. I wanted to have a full 16-hour day without fading to sleep in the middle of it. I wanted to go somewhere without having to take a preparatory nap first.

But ... patience. Small victories carry you through.

One day I became aware that I'd been standing for half an hour. It was a win; previously the myalgia had caused my legs to ache and go weak within five minutes. I had become Chair Guy. Now I saw I could walk without muscle aches and fatigue. Before, I could put on socks only by twisting into a pretzel and using stairs as an aid. Suddenly, well, almost suddenly, I could bend over and yank them on without falling down. It may seem perfectly normal to be able to put on socks, and it is. But you can lose what's ordinary and normal.

In aikido my body had crusted over and stratified to a point where I'd started to give up the falling, because my recalcitrant leg and abdominal muscles had become unwilling or unable to pull me back to a standing position. *Half is better than none*, I'd thought at the time, but it's not. Neither is half a cup of coffee or half a kiss. Aikido had become half depressing, after 45 years of joyful training, so my spirits began to lift, as with my body after a fall. It was awkward getting up, but I was standing.

"Air hunger" and excessive sweating are also common symptoms of late-stage or chronic Lyme. On the mat, I had become a huffing and puffing machine; in the dojo you could hear me over the thumps of people falling and rolling. I was a kind of soundtrack, but not in a good way. People would stop in the middle of a technique in the dead of winter with the room quite cold. "You're dripping—are you OK?" "It's a Lyme thing," I'd tell them, though seeing no subsequent flicker of recognition in their eyes. Never mind, it's my life and my embedded microbes.

The months of 2023 went by, and with each rip of the calendar page a piece of my former self returned. If my wife asked how I was feeling and I said, "Kinda normal," she knew I was improved. It was undeniable. I had gone from sleeping in three shirts topped with a hoodie (and under a down quilt) to just a cotton T-shirt and a cotton long-sleeved shirt over it. The increments of difference we can detect! The small plaques on my scalp that had first appeared only days before my foot neuropathy attacked 20 years ago seemed reduced by about half, with the largest barely there. I'd had chronic redness below my nose and around my chin almost since I could remember; now it was clear skin. The sweats and breathlessness upon exertion went drier and quieter. Not gone, but noticeably improved. After months and months, closer to "normal." Closer to the feelings and rhythms and responses of the person I used to be and still wanted to be.

I was able to go on drives farther than the little village where we live (town center is about three miles away). I was able to renew my driver's license (seriously, I couldn't navigate to the Department of Motor Vehicles before). I could go out to dinner with my wife and last until the end. I had the urge to go out into the world instead of fearing it. I no longer wanted to go back to sleep two hours after awakening.

Yes, that's the word; awakening. We don't realize our own natural vitality until it is at war with a pathogen, when all systems of the body are called into active duty and have no time for weekend leave, or for normal living.

I went to my PCP for an annual checkup in late summer of 2023, nine months after starting on botanicals. "Your eyes are brighter," she said. My vitals were fine (perfect blood pressure, average temperature, normal pulse), and the standard blood tests were in normal range all along the list. I was curious whether my complement C4a had changed along with the changes in my energy and feeling state. A quantitative change could reassure me that it wasn't all in my head, that the change was real and not just an inexplicable respite. She looked on her laptop to find the test on the standard lists they give doctors. "Oh," she said, "I'll have to write out an actual paper prescription for this; can't just do it electronically. It's not on the list, and a bit arcane."

That wasn't a surprise. The functional medicine doctors are plowing a different field than the allopathic docs. But at least the regular lab could run it. Back came the results in about a week, and there was a number that seemed in itself, even more than my returning vigor, to be the number that optimism wears on its team shirt. My C4a had gone from 4,500, nine times the high end of normal, down to 500, *within* the normal range.

Along with "feeling better," 500 landed like a kind of mainstream objective seal of approval for my constant dosing of herbal tinctures.

Yet I knew there was still more to go, farther on the road to full functioning normalcy. It was still a fragile state. I would still feel the old menu of symptoms if I got too little sleep, or played too hard in aikido or tennis, or ate badly, or was stressed out by relationships or the ups and downs of my investments. I was still like an old car, one that could get you there but would start to smoke at high revs.

2024:
A Twist on the Twist

Then something new crossed my path, a study from the University of Massachusetts published in summer of 2023. A graduate student in microbiology had had a bright idea. *Borrelia*, it had been found, got 100% of its energy (or nutrients) from a by-product of glycolysis, which is the body's processing of glucose for use in a variety of bodily functions (including brain activity). Since I'm not a scientist, I can't pretend to get too deep in the weeds here, but the logic of the UMass discovery goes something like this:

> *Borrelia burgdorferi*, the causative agent of Lyme disease, has a highly reduced genome and relies heavily on glycolysis for carbon metabolism. ...
>
> [G]lycolysis is the sole mechanism for *B. burgdorferi's* ATP [energy storage and release in cells] production. ... [T]he sole means by which *B. burgdorferi* can use pyruvate

> [make use of the energy that can be released through glycolysis] is by conversion to lactate via the enzyme lactate dehydrogenase (LDH). Thus, LDH is an essential metabolic linchpin for *B. burgdorferi*, and its inhibition could serve as an effective method for mitigating cell growth ... with minimal collateral effects on the host.

Without the LDH enzyme, *Borrelia* has no source of energy.

Wow, I thought, *what a concept*. Starve the buggers out while hitting them with something bactericidal at the same time!

The researchers, led by Adam Lynch, repurposed existing LDH inhibitors—some of which have already been used as adjuvant therapy in treating cancer—and used them for a set of in vitro experiments that were similar in character to those in the Johns Hopkins study I've cited earlier. Indeed, the results were similar, too, showing a dose-dependent annihilation of the *Borrelia* when the LDH enzyme was suppressed.

The existing commercial inhibitors, though, were daunting to me. They did not seem to be readily available, and some, at least, carried with them a variety of toxic effects. (One, gossypol, has even been considered as a method of male birth control because it is spermicidal!) So, jogging along the path of "natural" or low-harm products as I was, I sought out relatively benign substances that might have a similar effect. In fact, it turns out there are other LDH suppressors, such as berberine, a phytochemical found in the plants barberry and goldenseal, and ... wait for it ... good old vitamin C!

There's been much study of vitamin C and appropriate safe dosage, so I was able to get hold of some in liposomal form—the nutrient is embedded in tiny fat-like particles, enabling it to persist much longer in the body, unlike conventional vitamin C, which is excreted within 12 to 24 hours.

I added both berberine and 2000 mg of C to my armada of natural products, feeling fine about the safety of both (according to research studies) and knowing as well that C is purported to have a number of beneficial effects, including anti-inflammatory, antioxidant, and anticancer. It's even used by well-respected mainstream professionals as an IV infusion adjuvant therapy against cancer. So I'm like, yes, I want that. Who wouldn't?

We're into September of 2023 now, with my complement C4a already revealed by blood testing to be merely normal (down from "overdrive") and my general overall feeling, symptoms, and energy level improved. So I can't be sure if the vitamin C had any pointed effect—as I'd felt with *Cryptolepis* and knotweed when I first got started in December of 2022. But I did begin to feel sharper and clearer once I started the C. Subjectively, it felt like a polishing of metal that had been previously cleaned. Just subjective and only that? Placebo effect?

MY TAKEAWAYS AND A NOTION OF INFECTIOUS DISEASE

I recently had a conversation with a friend explaining my theory or notion of infection as:

1) an invasive microbe enters the bloodstream, or tissues, or central nervous system, and
2) various components of the immune system, mainly cytokines, go on the alert and are called into active duty.

But the immune system is crudely calibrated. Where a rifle might suffice, as often as not it uses a bazooka just to be sure. The symptoms we feel arise not from the microbe itself but from the reaction to it.

"You'd think the immune system would be balanced and only have a response that's appropriate, not more than is needed," said my friend, using simple logic and a sense that the body's ecosystem would naturally tend toward harmonious balance.

"Yes," I said, "you'd think. Obviously our inner health security system could use some design improvement."

Overcoming disease has to proceed on two fronts: killing the invader, plus modulating and demobilizing the armed forces mustered to destroy it. If the troops don't get the order to stand down, they can keep going long after their usefulness has waned, producing problems of their own making. It's called chronic inflammation.

The Johns Hopkins researchers started by acknowledging the anecdotal assertions of benefits from botanical treatments for Lyme. People have stories, and folks like Stephen Buhner have strong assertions, all of which the research team accepted as possible. "However, it is unclear whether the effect of the herb products is due to their direct antimicrobial activity or their effect on the host immune system." So they designed their study to remove the effect of the host's immune system or any other system, since in vitro there is no host. Just a neutral medium that itself can be tested and compared for any effect.

The big question, easy enough to miss in the dull scientific language this and nearly all other studies use to introduce their inspiration: Did they find that certain herbs actually killed or suppressed the *Borrelia*, or did those herbs improve the natural immune response by suppressing some of the inflammation that was actually the direct cause of symptoms? In other words, was there a magic bullet, or did the herbs create a more effective and accurate immune system by suppressing or modulating excessive inflammatory response to microbial invasion? By suppressing the host's cytokine cascade? Or was it both?

By removing the "host" from their tests and observations, they answered the first half of the question; selected botanicals, at the right dosages, *do* indeed terminate the Lyme-causing bacteria. But is that enough? By themselves? Out of the lab and in the body, there is surely more going on than just the bactericidal effect.

It seems apparent that if the immune system's actions are the cause of the symptoms that define disease, then you need to kill the invader, but you also need the immune system to do its job. What matters is that the immune system remain effective without going overboard. Inflammation causes the symptoms, the sickness, when the immune function *is too strong or lasts too long*. To counter this, anti-inflammatories are needed. Cue the botanicals. They are the balance the body needs, the balance that enables *both* bactericidal action and a controlled release of the immune system at the same time.

The plants in question may have dozens and dozens of active chemicals in them, and it might be that it is *combinations* of chemicals that make them effective. Can we separate killing bacteria from tranquilizing the immune reaction?

It would be interesting to find out. But why bother? We already know there are herbs that work well in vitro, and I'm here to tell you that at least in my case—one of the oldest documented cases of Lyme—they work in vivo too. And lots of lesser issues have been resolved by their anti-inflammatory effects.

Though in my working career I've often been opportunistic, here there's nothing to sell, no brand to build. I've simply become amazed and grateful that herbs could accomplish what industry's best and brightest drug developers can't—at least in this test case of one subject. I sincerely hope the information here will be helpful to fellow Lymies, people who love them, and the thousands and thousands of doctors, whatever their philosophy of healing, who need to know more about Lyme than they do.

2024:
My "Recipe"

In the end, there is only so much you can rely on from a story, albeit a true-life story, of just one individual. Having taken mountains of antibiotics during my Lyme years, including the 30-day intravenous infusion of what's purported to be the best in class, I found the mainstream allopathic direction to be lacking—almost completely lacking. Because the pharma companies had nothing to help, I went elsewhere with modest expectations at the time.

In the case of the particularly tough and resilient *Borrelia burgdorferi*, one is reluctant to use the word *cure*. Still, I'm feeling cured now, in mid-2024, though I remain alert for bacterial persistence and arousal. There were, after all, long periods when I felt fine before. Indeed, for the first 20 years, I didn't know I was chronically infected until it broke out in painful neuropathy. Still, I feel cured.

I'm not an expert, and not a celebrity, so there's no magic that should prompt you to listen to me. Nevertheless, here is what I did and what I do, for maintenance and as prophylaxis against a relapse. The list is unranked, because I honestly don't know which of the items could be as effective on their own. Here is my recipe (I don't use the pseudo-scientific term *protocol* because that's so last century):

- Hot baths or saunas, raising the body temperature to mild fever of 101.5°F or higher, daily
- Much more sleep than I would like: 9 to 11 hours seems like a healing dose.
- *Cryptolepis* tincture: Build to 2.0 mL dose several times daily.
- Japanese knotweed tincture: Build to 2 mL dose several times daily.
- *Artemisia* tincture: Build to 2 mL dose several times daily.
- Vitamin C (liposomal): 2000 mg daily
- Turmeric and ginger tincture: 4 mL dose several times daily (for general inflammation)
- Vigorous exercise
- Patience in sticking with all of it

If I had to choose just one herb, it would be ***Cryptolepis***, based on its performance against the several life stages of *Borrelia* in the Johns Hopkins study and its effect on me. Overall, everything in the list above is anti-inflammatory, in addition to whatever direct effect it may have on *Borrelia*, and may prompt a natural healing in various organs or systems beyond the specific needs of Lyme disease treatment.

My little recipe above is not medical advice and is not based on extensive double-blind clinical trials, as it should be to be credible. It's worth repeating that I am not a research scientist or a doctor, and I'm not offering medical advice. I just did what I did.

ABOUT THE AUTHOR

Lowell Miller is a writer, businessman, and artist, living in the Hudson Valley, NY.

Made in United States
Troutdale, OR
02/09/2025